Official Journal of the Skin Pharmacology Society (SPS) and
the International Society for Bioengineering and the Skin (ISBS)

Skin Pharmacology

Journal of Pharmacological and Biophysical Research

Incorporating 'Bioengineering and the Skin'

KARGER

Printed in Switzerland
on acid-free paper by
Thür AG Offsetdruck, Pratteln

Appears quarterly:
1 volume per year (4 issues)

Submission: Only original papers written in English should be sent to:

Prof. H. Schaefer
CIRD GALDERMA
Route des Lucioles
Sophia-Antipolis
F-06565 Valbonne Cedex (France)

or to

Dr. J. Serup
Leo Pharmaceutical Products
Department of Dermatological Research
55, Industriparken
DK-2750 Ballerup (Denmark)

Conditions: All manuscripts are subject to editorial review. Manuscripts are received with the explicit understanding that they are not under simultaneous consideration by any other publication. Submission of an article for publication implies the transfer of the copyright from the author to the publisher upon acceptance. Accepted papers become the permanent property of 'Skin Pharmacology' and may not be reproduced by any means, in whole or in part, without the written consent of the publisher. It is the author's responsibility to obtain permission to reproduce illustrations, tables, etc. from other publications. The journal consists of the following sections:

1. Editorials
2. Original Research Articles
3. Short Communications
4. Reviews
5. Research Forum and Letters to the Editor
6. SPS Transactions – News
7. Announcements

Short Communications: Authors may apply to have their paper treated as short communication. Condition for this is a brief definite report of important results. Final decision whether a paper will be published as a short communication will be made by the Editors. A publication time of three months after acceptance is intended.

Arrangement: Manuscripts should be submitted in triplicate *(with three sets of original illustrations),* typewritten double-spaced on one side of the paper, with a wide margin. They should comprise approximately 10 pages including figures, tables and references.

Title page: The first page of each paper should indicate the title (main title underlined), the authors' names, and the institute where the work was conducted. A short title for use as running head as well as the full address of the author to whom correspondence should be sent are also required.

Full address: The exact postal address complete with postal code must be given at the bottom of the title page. Please also supply Phone and Fax numbers.

Key words: For indexing purposes, a list of 3–10 key words in English is essential.

Abstract: Each paper needs an abstract in English of up to 10 lines. The abstract is of utmost importance. It should contain the following information: purpose of the study, procedures, results, conclusions and message of the paper.

Small type: Paragraphs which can or must be set in smaller type (case histories, methods, etc.) should be indicated with a 'p' (petit) in the margin on the left-hand side.

Footnotes: Avoid footnotes. When essential, they are numbered consecutively and typed at the foot of the appropriate page.

Tables and illustrations: Tables and illustrations (both numbered in Arabic numerals) should be prepared on separate sheets. Tables require a heading and figures a legend, also prepared on a separate sheet. For the reproduction of illustrations, only good drawings and original black and white glossy prints can be accepted; negatives or photocopies cannot be used. When possible, group several illustrations on one block for reproduction (max. size 144 × 196 mm) or provide crop marks. On the back of each illustration, indicate its number, the author's name, and 'top'. Color illustrations are reproduced at the author's expense.

References: In the text identify references by Arabic numerals [in square brackets]. Material submitted for publication but not yet accepted should be noted as 'unpublished data' and not be included in the reference list. The list of references should include only those publications which are cited in the text. Do not alphabetize; number references in the order in which they are first mentioned in the text. The surnames of the authors followed by initials should be given. There should be no punctuation other than a comma to separate the authors. Cite all authors, 'et al' is not sufficient. Abbreviate journal names according to the Index Medicus system. (Also see International Committee of Medical Journal Editors: Uniform requirements for manuscripts submitted to biomedical journals. Br Med J 1988;296: 401–405.)

Examples:

(a) Papers published in periodicals: Kauffman HF, van der Heide S, Beaumont F, Blok H, de Vries K: Class-specific antibody determination against *Aspergillus fumigatus* by means of the enzyme-linked immunosorbent assay. III. Comparative study: IgG, IgA, IgM ELISA titers, precipitating antibodies and IgE binding after fractionation of the antigen. Int Arch Allergy Appl Immunol 1986;80:300–306.

(b) Monographs: Matthews DE, Farewell VT: Using and Understanding Medical Statistics. Basel, Karger, 1985.

(c) Edited books: Hardy WD Jr, Essex M: FeLV-induced feline acquired immune deficiency syndrome: A model for human AIDS; in Klein E (ed): Acquired Immunodeficiency Syndrome. Prog Allergy. Basel, Karger, 1986, vol 37, pp 353–376.

Further details: Authors may consult our leaflet 'Rules for the Preparation of Manuscripts', available on request from the Publisher, S. Karger AG, P.O. Box, CH-4009 Basel (Switzerland).

Galley proofs: Unless indicated otherwise, galley proofs are sent to the first-named author and should be returned with the least possible delay. Alterations made in galley proofs, other than the correction of printer's errors, are charged to the author. No page proofs are supplied.

Reprints: Order forms and a price list are sent with the galley proofs. Orders submitted after the issue is printed are subject to considerably higher prices. Allow five weeks from date of publication for delivery of reprints.

KARGER

General Information

Skin Pharmacology

Publication data: 'Skin Pharmacology' is published 4 times annually. Volume 5 with 4 issues appears in 1992.

Subscription rates: Subscriptions run for a full calendar year. Prices are given per volume, surface postage included.

Personal subscription:
SFr. 196.–, US$ 130.90.
(Must be in the name of, billed to, and paid by an individual. Order must be marked 'personal subscription'.)

Institutional subscription:
(Regular rate.) SFr. 280.–, US$ 187.00.

Members of the Skin Pharmacology Society; Society for Bioengineering and the Skin: Subscription included in membership fee.

Airmail postage: SFr. 25.–, US$ 20.00.
(Extra per volume.)

Microform subscription:
SFr. 140.–, US$ 93.50.
(Available exclusively to subscribers of the paper edition.)

Single issues and back volumes: Information on availability and prices can be obtained through the Publisher.

Subscription orders: Orders can be placed at agencies, bookstores, directly with the Publisher S. Karger AG, P.O. Box, CH – 4009 Basel (Switzerland) or with any of the following distributors:

Deutschland:
S. Karger GmbH, Lörracher Strasse 16A
Postfach, D-W-7800 Freiburg

France: Librairie Luginbühl
36, bd de Latour-Maubourg
F-75007 Paris

Great-Britain, Ireland:
S. Karger Publishers
11 Ravenscroft Road
Beckenham, Kent BR3 4TP

USA: S. Karger Publishers, Inc.
26 West Avon Road, P.O. Box 529
Farmington, CT 06085

India, Bangladesh, Sri Lanka:
S. Karger India Subscription Agency
B – 5/132 Safdarjung Enclave
New Delhi-110029

Japan: Katakura Libri, Inc.
36-9 Hongo 3-chome, Bunkyo-ku
Tokyo 113

Change of address: Both old and new address should be stated and sent to the subscription source.

Bibliographic indices: This journal is regularly listed in bibliographic services, including *Current Contents®*.

Advertising: Correspondence and rate requests should be addressed to the Publisher.

KARGER

October 14–16, 1992
Cleveland, Ohio

9th Annual Meeting of the Skin Pharmacology Society

Abstracts

and

October 19 and 20, 1992
Sendai, Japan

9th ISBS Meeting
The International Symposium on Bioengineering and the Skin

Abstracts

KARGER

S. Karger
Medical and Scientific Publishers
Basel · Freiburg · Paris · London
New York · New Delhi · Bangkok
Singapore · Tokyo · Sydney

Drug Dosage
The authors and the publisher have exerted every effort to ensure that drug selection and dosage set forth in this text are in accord with current recommendations and practice at the time of publication. However, in view of ongoing research, changes in government regulations, and the constant flow of information relating to drug therapy and drug reactions, the reader is urged to check the package insert for each drug for any change in indications and dosage and for added warnings and precautions. This is particularly important when the recommended agent is a new and/or infrequently employed drug.

Printed in Switzerland on acid-free paper by
Thür AG Offsetdruck, Pratteln
ISBN 3-8055-5692-6

Contents

Skin Pharmacol 1992;5:193–207

October 14–16, 1992
Stouffer Tower City
Plaza Hotel
Cleveland, Ohio (USA)

9th Annual Meeting of the Skin Pharmacology Society

Abstracts

1

Biotransformation of Leukotriene A_4 to Leukotriene C_4 by Affinity-Purified Glutathione S-Transferase from Rat Skin

R. Agarwal, H. Raza, D.R. Bickers, H. Mukhtar
Department of Dermatology, Case Western Reserve University, and VA Medical Center, Cleveland, Ohio, USA

Leukotrienes (LTs) constitute a group of oxygenated metabolites of arachidonic acid (AA) with biological activity related to hypersensitivity and inflammation. Biosynthesis of LT proceeds via unstable intermediate LTA_4 formed by the 5-lipoxygenase pathway of AA metabolism. A major route of LTA_4 biotransformation is conjugation of its epoxy group with reduced glutathione (GSH) leading to the formation of LTC_4. In spite of the fact that the skin is major site of inflammation and is susceptible to various allergic and anaphylactic reactions mediated by the cysteine-containing LTs, the ability of glutathione S-transferase (GSTs) to catalyze the conjugation of LTA_4 to LTC_4 in this tissue has not been investigated. Recently, we have shown evidence for multiple isozymes of GSTs in human and rodent skin. In the present study we have purified GST from rat skin cytosol by GSH-agarose affinity chromatography and showed that this preparation effectively mediates the conjugation of GSH with LTA_4-methyl ester resulting in the formation of LTC_4-methyl ester. Affinity-purified GST also exhibited several-fold increase in the specific activity of enzyme with 1-chloro-2,4-dinitrobenzene (55-fold), ethacrynic acid (67-fold) and LTA_4-methyl ester (12-fold) as substrates, as compared to crude cytosol. Western blot analysis of the affinity-purified GST indicated predominant expression of GST Pi isozyme followed by Mu and Alpha. The conjugation of LTA_4-methyl ester to LTC_4-methyl ester by affinity-purified GST was an enzymatic process with a K_m of 13.8 μM and V_{max} of 250 pmol/min/mg protein under optimal assay conditions. The formation of LTC_4-methyl ester was established by its radioactivity profile on HPLC and absorption spectroscopy. These results suggest that in addition to xenobiotic metabolism, cutaneous GSTs may also be capable of metabolizing physiological substrates such as LTA_4.

2

Platelet-Activating Factor (PAF) and Lyso-PAF in Inflamed Skin

R.M. Barr, M.R. Judge, A.I. Mallet, F. Lawlor, P.F. Courtney, A. Kobza Black, R. Barlow, M.W. Greaves
St. John's Institute of Dermatology, London, UK

PAF, but not lyso-PAF, is pro-inflammatory, but the extent of PAF synthesis in skin and its contribution to inflammation is unclear. As lyso-PAF is both the precursor and hydrolysis product of PAF, we assayed PAF and lyso-PAF in inflamed skin. Suction blister fluids were obtained from skin of healthy volunteers and patients with delayed pressure urticaria (DPU) or mastocytosis. Exudates were collected from abraded skin of normal subjects and patients with psoriasis or allergic dermatitis to nickel. PAF and lyso-PAF were assayed by GC-MS. PAF concentrations in blister fluid from normal healthy skin were 1.86 ± 0.92 nM, (mean ± SEM), from DPU before and 6 h after pressure stimulation 1.41 ± 0.32 and 1.76 ± 0.32, respectively;

uninvolved and lesional mastocytosis, 1.58 ± 0.31 and 1.52 ± 0.27, respectively, were similar. Mean lyso-PAF concentrations, range 160–280 n*M*, also showed no differences between these groups. PAF levels in abrasion exudates of normal skin, uninvolved and lesional psoriatic skin, and 96-hour nickel dermatitis were within the range 0.3–0.6 pmol/abrasion. Lyso-PAF was lower in uninvolved than in lesional psoriatic skin, 3.1 ± 0.43 and 9.5 ± 1.9 pmol/abrasion. Lyso-PAF was lower in uninvolved than in lesional psoriatic skin, 3.1 ± 0.43 and 9.5 ± 1.9 pmol/abrasion ($p < 0.05$), respectively. The corticosteroid clobetasol propionate (0.05% applied occluded for 72 h on normal skin) reduced lyso-PAF in blister fluid to 152 ± 24 compared with 230 ± 42 n*M* for the control sites ($p < 0.05$). PAF was reduced in 6/8 subjects by the steroid, but the decrease was not significant. We conclude that if PAF is a significant mediator in inflamed skin, it may remain associated with the synthesising cell or acts in its immediate proximity.

3

The Pro-Proliferative Effects of Vasoactive Peptides on Human Dermal Microvascular and Large Vessel Endothelium

Helen A. Bull[a], *Diane Abbot*[a], *Paul M. Brickell*[b], *Pauline M. Dowd*[a]
Departments of [a] Dermatology and [b] Biochemistry, University College and Middlesex School of Medicine, The Middlesex Hospital, London, UK

Vasoactive peptides such as calcitonin gene-related peptide (CGRP) and endothelin-1 (ET-1) may modulate vascular endothelial cell responses at sites of tissue injury and hence have a trophic and cell-regulatory role. We have therefore investigated (i) the effect of these peptides on DNA replication, serine protease activity and expression of the extracellular matrix protein von Willebrand factor protein (vWF) in both microvascular human dermal microvascular endothelial cells (HDMEC) and large vessel human umbilical vein endothelial cells (HUVEC) and (ii) the potential role of protein tyrosine phosphorylation in post-receptor signalling mechanisms in these processes. CGRP and ET-1 (10^{-14} to 10^{-6} *M*) increased incorporation of bromodeoxyuridine (BrdU) in HDMEC but only CGRP increased BrdU incorporation in HUVEC. The response curves were bell-shaped with a significant increase induced in HDMEC by 10^{-11} to 10^{-10} *M* βCGRP and 10^{-12} to 10^{-11} *M* ET-1 and in HUVEC by 10^{-11} to 10^{-10} *M* βCGRP and 10^{-11} *M* αCGRP. Both β CGRP (10^{-13} to 10^{-11} *M*), αCGRP (10^{-14} *M*) and ET-1 (10^{-10} to 10^{-8} *M*) significantly increased serine protease activity in HUVEC ($n = 4$, $p < 0.05$) but not in HDMEC whilst neither peptide altered vWF expression in either HDMEC or HUVEC. Western blots of protein extracts prepared from HDMEC and HUVEC were probed with anti-phosphotyrosine antibodies. Phsophotyrosine-containing proteins were evident in unstimulated HDMEC and HUVEC, but there was no change in the pattern of tyrosine phosphorylation in either cell type incubated with 10^{-11} *M* βCGRP or 10^{-11} *M* ET-1 for 22 h. These data demonstrate that CGRP and ET-1 potentiate DNA replication in HDMEC but have no effect on other angiogenic responses. In HUVEC, CGRP potentiates DNA replication and both CGRP and ET-1 increse serine protease activity. Peptide-induced increase in DNA replication is not associated with changes in the phosphotyrosine protein profile in either HUVEC or HDMEC. The proproliferative effects of these peptides in HDMEC further highlight the importance of these peptides in the maintenance of cutaneous microvascular homoeostasis.

4

Modification of Neutrophil Function by Naftifine

T.S. Choi, B.A. Solomon, W.L. Lee, S.C. Geen, A.R. Shalita
Department of Dermatology, SUNY Health Science Center at Brooklyn, Brooklyn, N.Y., USA

Naftifine (NF), a topical antimycotic agent, is highly active in vitro and in vivo against a wide range of pathogenic fungi. When added to polymorphonuclear leukocytes (PMNs), NF inhibited PMN chemotaxis (CT). Following stimulation with zymosan-activated serum or f-met-leu-phe, a maximum of 85–97% of the PMNs (preincubation with NF for 2–30 min at 1–125 μg/ml at 37 °C) exhibited easily detectable membrane ruffling, and polarity. In contrast, no NF-treated PMN exhibited such chemotactic factor-induced shape changes. Our results indicated NF also inhibits PMN respiratory burst (RB) activity in an irreversible dose-dependent and time-independent manner, as evaluatd by PMN chemiluminescence (emission of photons from oxygen radical) and superoxide (O_2^-) production. In addition to inhibiting CT and RB activity, NF (at 5–20 µg/ml) significantly inhibited adherence of PMNs to endothelial monolayers ($p < 0.01–0.001$) as assessed by dye uptake assay. In conclusion, NF can alter the membrane-related responses on human PMN; this alteration may be associated with a change in PMN morphology. The data collectively document morphological and functional differences between normal and NF-treated PMNs as determined by stimulus-specific Cl and O_2^- generation and chemotactic factor-induced membrane shape change. Such differences may account, in part, for its efficacy in inflammatory skin diseases.

5

15-Lipoxygenase Expression in Keratinocytes

B.M. Czarnetzki[a], *S. Binting*[a], *T. Rosenbach*[a], *P. Ludwig*[b], *C. Hiebsch*[b], *B. Thiele*[b], *T. Schewe*[b]
[a] Department of Dermatology, Clinical Immunology, and Asthma, UKRV, FU Berlin, and [b] Institute of Biochemistry, Charité, Humboldt University, Berlin, FRG

Keratinocytes have been reported to produce 15-HETE, but the presence of 15-lipoxygenase (15-LOX) has not been demonstated so far. In order to investigate the role of 15-LOX in keratinocyte differentiation, HaCaT keratinocytes were examined for 15-LOX activity, 15-LOX protein, and 15-LOX mRNA by means of chiral phase HPLC, Western and Northern blot techniques. The results suggest an expression of 15-LOX protein in HaCaT keratinocytes and normal human keratinocytes. Immunohistochemical staining of skin specimens revealed a stronger staining pattern in basal keratinocytes than in differentiated keratinocytes. Chiral phase analysis of 15-HETE generated by HaCaT keratinocytes showed at least in part a 15-LOX-specific conversion of arachidonic acid. Inhibition of 15-LOX by the specific inhibitor BAF 3162 suppressed keratinocte differentiation as measured by involucrin formation. These results suggest that keratinocytes possess 15-LOX activity and that 15-LOX may play a role in keratinocyte differentiation.

6

Regulation of the Immune Response to Dimethylbenz(a)anthracene Is Governed By Genes within the Major Histocompatibility Complex and at the Ah Receptor Locus

C.A. Elmets, M. Athar, S.L. Zaidi, H. Mukhtar
Department of Dermatology, Case Western Reserve University, Cleveland, Ohio, USA

In previous studies, we have shown that the polyaromatic hydrocarbon carcinogen dimethylbenz(a)anthracene (DMBA) is capable of eliciting a potent allergic contact hypersensitivity response when applied to the skin of C3H mice. The genetic requirements for the development of this type of reaction in mice were investigated in this study. Many of the biological effects of DMBA require that it first be metabolized by enzymes induced by the Ah receptor. Initial studies were therefore performed to evaluate the development of DMBA contact hypersensitivity in Ah receptor-negative strains of mice. All such strains tested (DBA/2, AKR/J, SJL/J) failed to develop a response, indicating that the Ah receptor was necessary for development of contact hypersensitivity to DMBA. Although most Ah receptor-positive strains of mice did develop DMBA contact hypersensitivity, some (C57Bl/6, C57Bl/10) did not. As a result, experiments were conducted to determine if genes within the murine major histocompatibility complex represented a second restriction element for DMBA contact hypersensitivity. When Ah receptor-positive, MHC-congenic mice were evaluated, a substantially greater DMBA contact hypersensitivity response was observed in $H\text{-}2^k$ (C3H, B10.BR) and $H\text{-}2^a$ (A/J, B10.A(1R), B10.A) than in $H\text{-}2^s$ (B10.S, A.SW) or $H\text{-}2^b$ (C57Bl/10, C57Bl/6, A.BY, C3H.SW) haplotype mice. Although C57Bl/6 (Ah receptor-positive, $H\text{-}2^b$ haplotype) and AKR (Ah receptor-negative, $H\text{-}2^k$ haplotype) failed to develop a contact hypersensitivity response, C57Bl/6 × AKR F_1 hybrids could be sensitized to DMBA, indicating that gene complementation had occurred. Finally, responding C3H mice were compared with nonresponding C3H.SW mice for their susceptibility to DMBA-induced skin cancer. C3H mice developed significantly fewer tumors than did C3H.SW mice. The results indicate that the development of contact hypersensitivity to DMBA is governed by genes within the major histocompatibility complex and at the Ah receptor locus. Moreover, strain differences in the capacity to develop DMBA contact hypersensitivity parallel differences in the resistance of these strains to DMBA-induced skin tumors.

7

A Double-Blind, Parallel-Group Study of the Efficacy and Safety of Ammonium Lactate 12% Lotion in the Treatment of Photodamaged Skin

J.R. Gibson[a], *V. Stevens*[a], *J. Leyden*[b], *M.J. Grove*[b], *N. Lowe*[c], *T. Bourget*[c], *J. Weiss*[d], *B. Shavin*[d]
[a] Bristol-Myers Squibb PRI, Buffalo, N.Y., USA; [b] KGL, Inc., Philadelphia, Pa., USA; [c] Skin Research Foundation, Santa Monica, Calif., USA; [d] Gwinnett Clinical Research Center, Snellville, Ga., USA

The purpose of this work was to evaluate ammonium lactate 12% lotion (Lac-Hydrin® 12% Lotion, Westwood-Squibb) in the treatment of photodamaged skin. The study had a double-blind, randomized, parallel-group design. Male and female subjects of 35 years or older with photodamage of the face and forearms of at leasts moderate severity (grade 4 on a 0–8 scale) were enrolled. The test agent or its vehicle were applied twice daily for 6 months and clinical evaluations were conducted regularly throughout the treatment period. Overall severity and ten individual characteristics of photodamage were graded using a 0–8 scale. In addition, the physician's and the patient's global evaluation of improvement/worsening were independently recorded. The face and the forearms were assessed separately. High-quality, standardized photographs and skin surface replicas from the periorbital area were obtained. Ninety subjects were enrolled and they all yielded evaluable data. Results indicated that ammonium lactate 12% lotion could be statistically significantly separated from its vehicle in terms of efficacy from as early as 4 weeks of treatment. By 16 weeks of therapy, approximately 90% of subjects using the active agent had a slight or moderate improvement in the overall severity of their condition compared with less than 20% of those using vehicle. The overall trend was for progressive improvement to occur, in those parameters which responded such as fine wrinkling, throughout the treatment period. Both the active agent and its vehicle were well tolerated. It is concluded that ammonium lactate 12% lotion is superior to its vehicle in the treatment of photodamaged skin. The degree of benefit is generally in the slight to moderate range and it is speculated that higher concentrations may yield an even more effective therapeutic modality which should still retain a very acceptable safety profile.

8

A Study of Immunoreactive Nerves in Vibration White Finger

P.C. Goldsmith, *C.B. Bunker*[a], *T.A. Leslie*[a], *G. Terenghi*[b], *F. Abadia Molina*[b], *J. Polak*[b], *Pauline M. Dowd*[a]
[a] Department of Dermatology, University College and Middlesex School of Medicine, [b] Department of Histochemistry, The Royal Postgraduate Medical School, Hammersmith Hospital, London, UK

Vibration white finger (VWF) or Raynaud's phenomenon (RP) of occupational origin is the episodic blanching of the fingers in response to cold in those who work with hand-held vibrating tools. Unlike RP persistent paresthesiae and pain are common in the hands and arms and those with the disorder are predominantly male. It is a financially compensatable industrial disorder for which there is no diagnostic test. Patients with primary RP and RP secondary to systemic sclerosis have been shown to have a deficiency of the powerful vasodilator and sensory neuropeptide calcitonin gene-related peptide (CGRP) and normal amounts of the vasoconstrictor endothelin-1 (ET-1) in the digital cutaneous microvasculature. We therefore investigated the distribution of immunoreactive CGRP and ET-1 in the microvasculature in digital skin of patients with VWF. Digital cutaneous biopsies were taken from the dorsal aspect of the proximal phalanx in 16 men with VWF (mean age 52, range 30–72) and in 26 control male manual workers without a history of exposure to vibrating machinery (mean age 43, range 26–62) from matched digital sites. The diagnosis of VWF as made on occupational history, a characteristic history of attacks of RP and paraesthesiae with the absence of trophic changes and sclerodactyly. Clinical examination and investigations performed excluded known associated diseases. The biopsies were fixed in Zamboni's fixative, transferred to phosphate-buffered saline, cryostat blocks were prepared and 10-μm sections were cut. Immunostaining was carried out according to the indirect immunofluorescence method with antisera to protein gene product 9.5 (PGP 9.5 is a pan-neuronal marker), CGRP and ET-1. A marked depletion of both PGP 9.5 and CGRP immunoreactive nerve fibres was found in the epidermis and papillary dermis in the digital biopsies from the VWF patients when compared to the control group. The ET-1 staining was the same in both groups. These findings represent a less selective loss of immunoreactive nerve fibres than occurred in primary and secondary RP. This different pattern of neuronal loss may reflect the exogenous nature of the aetiology of the condition and is consistent with both a pathogenetic role in the vasodilator/vasoconstrictor imbalance and in the persistent sensory abnormalities characterising this condition. They also provide a diagnostic histological test for VWF.

9

Interaction of MK886, a Novel Leukotriene Biosynthesis Inhibitor, with Protein Kinase C

Lutz Hegemann, Christine Hann, Guy F. Webster, Jouni Uitto
Department of Dermatology, Thomas Jefferson University, Philadelphia, Pa., USA

Leukotrienes have been shown to be associated with several inflammatory diseases, including psoriasis. Therefore, MK886, a potent inhibitor of leukotriene biosynthesis with a novel mechanism of action has been suggested for the treatment of psoriasis. However, in recent clinical trials, the drug was found not to exert therapeutic effects in psoriasis. In the present study, we investigated the effects of MK886 on protein kinase C (PKC), a key enzyme in cellular signal transduction, which plays an important role in the pathophysiology of psoriasis. The drug was found to stimulate PKC activity in a dose-dependent manner. Further investigation of the mechanism of PKC stimulation and comparison to known PKC activators, such as phorbol esters, revealed the following results: MK886- and phorbol ester-stimulated enzyme activity was inhibited by known PKC inhibitors with identical potency. In contrast to other activators, MK886 did not require the presence of phospholipids to stimulate PKC. Since no effects of MK886 on the catalytic domain of PKC were observed, our data provide strong evidence that MK886 stimulates PKC by a novel mechanism of action. We have previously reported that antipsoriatic drugs, such as anthralin, inhibit PKC, and there is evidence that inhibition of PKC might be of therapeutic value in the treatment of psoriasis. Therefore, our finding that MK886 stimulates PKC activity might account for the lack of the drug's therapeutic efficacy and might explain some of the side effects observed in clinical trials.

10

Multiple Inducible Cytochrome P450 Isozymes in Human Epidermal Keratinocytes

F.K. Jugert, R. Agarwal, S. Frankenberg, H. Junginger, D.R. Bickers, H. Mukhtar, H.F. Merk
Departments of Dermatology, University of Cologne, FRG, and Case Western Reserve University, Cleveland, Ohio, USA

Skin is a major interface between the body and the environment. It has been shown that skin possesses an important biochemical barrier against its environment, besides its physicochemical and immunochemical properties. Several studies have shown that skin possesses inducible cytochrome P450 (P450), which in addition to its role in the elimination of xenobiotics plays a role in the causation of skin disorders including contact sensitization and carcinogenesis, induced by drugs and environmental agents. In this study we investigated the effect of different chemicals, which are known to induce P450 isozymes in the liver, on the catalytic activities of different P450 isozymes in cultured human keratinocytes (HK). Proliferating HK were incubated for 48 h with inducing agents; microsomes were prepared and the monooxygenase activities were determined. Compared to vehicle-treated controls, the incubation of HK with benz(a)anthracene resulted in a 8- and 20-fold increase in the P4501A1-depencent acrylhydrocarbon hydroxylase and 7-ethoxyresorufin O-deethylase activities, respectively. Similarly, treatment with phenobarbital enhanced the P4502B1-dependent 7-pentoxyresorufin O-deethylase activity by 3.6-fold. Ethanol treatment of HK resulted in a 1.8-fold increase in the P4502E1-dependent paranitrophenol hydroxylase activity. Cyclosporine and dexamethasone induced the P4503A-dependent erythromycin N-demethylase activity by 2.7- and 2.4-fold, respectively. Our data indicate that treatment of HK with several inducers of P450 results in the enhanced activity of at least four subfamilies of three P450 gene families. These results verify that HK contain multiple inducible P450 isozymes capable of participating in the metabolism of carcinogens, solvents and drugs.

11

Induction of Cytochrome P450 Subfamilies 1A, 2B, 2E and 3A in Murine Skin by Dexamethasone

Frank K. Jugert, Rajesh Agarwal, David R. Bickers, Hans F. Merk, Hasan Mukhtar
Departments of Dermatology, University of Cologne, FRG, and Case Western Reserve University, Cleveland, Ohio, USA

Medications containing dexamethasone (DEX) are widely used as topical agents in dermatologic practice. Systemic administration of DEX to animals is known to result in the induction of multiple forms of cytochrome P450 (P450) isozymes in liver. In this study the effect of topical application of DEX to NMRI and SENCAR mice on P450-dependent monooxygenase activities and on P450 isozyme expression in cutaneous microsomes was assessed. Compared to control animals, skin application of DEX to mice resulted in varying degrees of induction of 7-ethoxyresorufin O-deethylase, 7-pentoxyresorufin O-deethylase, para-nitrophenol hydroxylase and erythromycin N-demethylase, the monooxygenases that are preferentially catalyzed by P450 isoenzymes 1A, 2B, 2E and 3A, respectively. In additional experiments, Western blotting with highly specific antibodies was used to assess the P450 isozyme induction response. Similar to catalytic activities, as compared to control animals, cutaneous microsomes obtained from DEX-treated mice showed an increased immunoreactivity with monoclonal and/or polyclonal antibodies directed against hepatic microsomal P450 1A, 2B, 2E and 3A. Dot-Blot hybridization of mRNA with specific primers for P450 1A and 2E showed increased reactivity in DEX-treated animals as compared to controls. These data further confirmed that application of DEX to murine skin results in increased P450 1A and 2E gene message. The results of our study show that the application of DEX to murine skin results in the induction of multiple P450 isozymes, which may participate in the metabolism of drugs such as glucocorticoids.

12

Skin Cancer Chemoprevention by Green Tea Polyphenols

S.K. Katiyar, R. Agarwal, G.S. Wood, H. Mukhtar
Department of Dermatology, Case Western Reserve University, and VAMC, Cleveland, Ohio,USA

Next to water, tea from *Camellia sinensis* is the most popular and common beverage in the world. In our prior studies, we have shown that oral feeding or topical application of polyphenolic fraction isolated from green tea (GTP) protects against chemical- as well as UVB radiation-induced carcinogenesis in murine skin [Carcinogenesis 1989;10:441–445, 1991;12: 1527–1530]. In the present study the effect of skin application of GTP to SENCAR mice on 12-O-tetradecanoylphorbol-13-acetate (TPA)-induced epidermal inflammation and hyperplasia, ornithine decarboxylase (ODC), cyclooxygenase and lipoxygenase activities was assessed. Prior application of GTP to mouse skin resulted in respectively 31–46% and 30–43% inhibition of TPA-induced epidermal inflammation and hyperplasia. Preapplication of GTP also resulted in inhibition of TPA-induced epidermal ODC activity in a dose-dependent manner. Similarly, as quantitated by the formation of PGE_2, $PGF_{2\alpha}$ and PGD_2, and 12/15 HETE, 8-HETE and 5-HETE metabolites from respectively cyclooxygenase- and lipoxygenase-catalyzed metabolism of arachidonic acid, preapplication of GTP also resulted in the inhibition of TPA-induced activity of these two enzymes. When assessed in an antitumor promotion protocol in 7, 12-dimethylbenz[α]anthracene-initiated SENCAR mouse skin, application of GTP (1–24 mg/application/animal) 30 min prior to that of TPA resulted in significant protection against skin tumor promotion. At doses of 1 and 24 mg GTP, more than 30% and almost complete protection, respectively, was observed. The results of the present study suggest that GTP possesses anti-skin tumor-promoting effects, and that the mechanism of such effects involves inhibition of tumor promoter-induced epidermal inflammation, hyperplasia, and ODC, cyclooxygenase and lipoxygenase activities. Further studies are in progress to define which component present in GTP is responsible for its cancer chemopreventive effects.

13

Basal Cell Carcinoma: Diminished Expression of Hemidesmosome-Associated Components

N.J. Korman, S. Hrabovsky
Department of Dermatology, Case Western Reserve University, Cleveland, Ohio, USA

Basal cell carcinoma (BCC) of the skin is the most commonly diagnosed cancer in the United States. Although these tumors are usually amenable to conservative therapy, a significant proportion of BCCs become locally aggressive with extensive tissue invasion. Specific antigenic defects in the basement membrane (BM) surrounding BCC tumor islands have been identified. Prior studies have shown absent or diminished expression of bullous pemphigoid antigen (BPA), a protein associated with hemidesmosomes. In the present study our aim was to determine whether there are abnormalities of other hemidesmosomal associated components in BCCs. Fresh BCCs were obtained from Moh's surgery specimens and frozen sections of these tumors were studied using fluorescein-labelled antibodies. Components analyzed include: (1) the 230 kD BPA, (2) the α_6 and β_4 subunits of the α_6 β_4 integrin, and (3) epiligrin. Seventeen papulonodular BCCs had marked diminution in the 230-kD BPA and in both the α_6 and β_4 subunits of α_6 β_4 integrin compared to overlying normal epidermal BM. All 8 papulonodular BCCs studied demonstrated markedly decreased levels of epiligrin in the tumor tissue compared to the overlying normal epidermal BM. These findings demonstrate significant defects in several hemidesmosome-associated components found in BCCs and suggest that these BM abnormalities may play a role in BCC invasion.

14

Capsaicin Modulates the Cutaneous Response to Endothelin-1

T.A. Leslie[a], N. Hayes[b], N.J. Levell[a], J.C. Foreman[b], P.M. Dowd[a]
Departments of [a] Dermatology and [b] Pharmacology, University College and Middlesex School of Medicine, London, UK

Endothelin-1 (ET-1), an endothelial cell-derived peptide, elicits intense vasoconstriction after intradermal injection and also causes a vasodilatation peripheral to the pallor, possibly mediated by peptidergic neuronal activity. ET-1 has been implicated in the pathophysiology of Raynauds phenomenon (RP) [Lancet 1990;336:1144–1147]. A reduction of calcitonin gene-related peptide (CGRP) fibres in digital skin of patients with RP has been demonstrated, but vascular responses are normal to intradermal CGRP [Lancet 1990;336:1530–1533]. We have (1) evaluated the role of peptidergic nerves in the control of digital cutaneous blood flow (DCBF), (2) determined whether neuropeptide depletion with capsaicin pretreatment leads to a reduction of DCBF as occurs in RP and (3) assessed the effect of topical capsaicin on the response to intradermal injection of ET-1. Capsaicin ointment (2% w/v) was applied under occlusion for 3 days to the middle digit of a hand in 11 normal subjects. On the 4th day intradermal injections of 25 μl of 2.5 μM ET-1 (distal phalanx) or normal saline (proximal phalanx) were made on the capsaicin-pretreated finger and also on an untreated finger. The areas of pallor and erythema were measured by planimetry and DCBF by laser Doppler flowmetry (LDF) at 2, 10 and 20 min after injection at 20 °C. We have shown that digital pretreatment with topical capsaicin for 3 days results in a significant reduction in the erythema response to ET-1 measured by LDF (%) (Wilcoxon: $p < 0.05$) and by planimetry (mm^2) (Wilcoxon: $p < 0.05$) compared to the control digits at each time point. The planimetry measurements in capsaicin-pretreated digits for ET-1-induced pallor also showed a significant decrease (Wilcoxon $p < 0.05$) at each time point. The baseline LDF measurements of capsaicin-pretreated and normal digits at the ET-1 and saline sites did not differ significantly. These results suggest that peptidergic nerves are involved in mediating the erythema response induced by ET-1. Capsaicin pretreatment of normal digits results in a reduction of DCBF and ET-1 flare size as occurs in patients with RP. The results support a role for the peptidergic nervous system in controlling blood flow in normal digital skin, and a defect in peptidergic neuronal control of blood flow in RP. The reduction in pallor size in capsaicin-pretreated digits could indicate that pallor is partly neurogenic or that capsaicin has a direct effect on the microvasculature.

15

Clearance of Lichen Planus with Very Low Dose Cyclosporin A

Nicholas J. Levell, Janet M. Marks
Dermatology Department, Newcastle upon Tyne, UK

Clearance of lichen planus (LP) with 3–5 mg/kg daily of cylcosporin (CsA) has been described. There is evidence that a much smaller systemic dose may be effective in oral LP, as the response described in some studies of high doses of topical CsA given as a mouthwash may have been due to systemic absorption of a small amount of the mouthwash. We have treated 4 patients with severe symptomatic cutaneous LP (2 of whom also had oral lesions) unresponsive to topical corticosteroids, with 1 mg/kg/day CsA. They were assessed 2-weekly and the dose increased by 50 mg daily every 4 weeks until clearance. Two patients cleared after 4 weeks on 1 mg/kg/day, 1 after 6 weeks on doses up to 2 mg/kg/day and 1 after 2.5 weeks on doses up to 2.5 mg/kg/day. Improvement was seen in some patients taking 1 mg/kg/day when blood levels of CsA were undetectable, but all patients had detectable blood levels of CsA (38–95 ng/ml) at clearance. No changes in blood pressure, hepatic or renal function were detected. In these patients LP cleared with < 50% of the oral dose and 3–10% of the dose of mouthwash used in previous studies. This supports our suggestion that the effect of the mouthwash may have been systemic. Controlled studies of the efficacy and toxicity of very low doses of CsA in LP should be made.

16

The Effect of Terbinafine on the Pharmacokinetics of Cyclosporin in vivo

C.C. Long[a], *S.A. Hill*[a], *R.C. Thomas*[a], *D.W. Holt*[b], *A.Y. Finlay*[a]
[a] Department of Dermatology, University of Wales College of Medicine, Cardiff, Wales;
[b] St. George's Hospital, London, UK

Cyclosporin is largely metabolised by hepatic cytochrome P450 enzymes, and azole drugs which inhibit cytochrome P450 may cause cyclosporin toxicity. The allylamine terbinafine binds to a small subfraction of hepatic cytochrome P450 in type I fashion and has no effect upon hepatic metabolism of cyclosporin in vitro [Back D, Tjia J: Br J Clin Pharmacol 1991;32:624–626]. The purpose of this study was to dermine whether oral terbinafine alters the pharmacokinetics of oral cyclosporin in vivo. Twenty male volunteers (age 19–24 years) were randomly allocated to two groups. The first group received 3 single oral doses of cyclosporin 300 mg at intervals of 21 days. The 2nd and 3rd doses of cyclosporin were preceded by a 6-day course of oral terbinafine 250 mg mane. A further 250 mg of terbinafine was taken with the 2nd and 3rd doses of cyclosporin. Blood levels of cyclosporin and terbinafine were monitored for 36 h after each dose. The second group received a 7-day course of terbinafine 250 mg mane. On the 7th day a single dose of cyclosporin 300 mg was taken together with the terbinafine. Blood levels of both cyclosporin and terbinafine were monitored for 36 h. Two further single doses of cyclosporin 300 mg were given at intervals of 2 weeks and the cyclosporin levels again monitored. In both groups each cyclosporin dose was preceded by an 8-hour fast. The mean peak blood concentration of cyclosporin (C_{max}) when taken alone was 958.4 µg/l (SD 248), and 821.6 (SD 251) when taken with terbinafine. The mean area under the curve (AUC) for cyclosporin was 4,207 µg/l/h (SD 1,123) when taken alone and 3,664.6 (SD 886) when taken with terbinafine. The mean absorption half-life for cyclosporin when taken alone was 0.29 h (SD 0.08), and 0.33 (SD 0.14) when taken with terbinafine. The mean time of maximum concentration (T_{max}) and elimination half-life of cyclosporin were unaltered by terbinafine. The results show a slight (12%) decrease in the mean AUC when cyclosporin is taken with terbinafine, the explanation for this is unclear. There is no evidence of any interaction likely to cause an increase in cyclosporin levels with resultant toxicity.

of individual lipids do not facilitate barrier recovery; instead, a proper mixture of cholesterol, fatty acids, and ceramides is required for barrier homeostasis, and (2) incomplete mixtures of topical lipids inhibit barrier recovery at the level of the lamellar body, resulting in the formation of abnormal intercellular membrane bilayers, abnormalities which are corrected with provision of a complete lipid mixture.

17

The Specific Lipid Requirements for Stratum Corneum Barrier Function. I. Effects of Individual vs. Mixtures of Lipids on Barrier Recovery in Acetone-Treated Murine Skin

Man Mao-Qiang, Kenneth R. Feingold, Peter M. Elias
Dermatology and Metabolism Sections, VAMC, San Francisco, Calif., USA

After permeability barrier disruption with acetone, transepidermal water loss rates normalize over 24 h as a result of both secretion of prestored lipid and accelerated lipid synthesis. Whereas previous studies have shown the importance of cholesterol, fatty acid and sphingolipid synthesis for barrier homeostasis, applications of certain of these key lipids individually can aggravate rather than improve barrier function. Hence, we asked whether these lipids need to be applied in a correct mixture to produce normal barrier recovery in acetone-treated hairless mouse skin. Fatty acids and ceramides alone, complex derivatives of the individual lipids (cholesterol esters, acylceramides, and cerebrosides), as well as incomplete lipid mixtures (fatty acids plus ceramides, cholesterol plus fatty acids, or cholesterol plus ceramides) impaired barrier recovery after topical application. In contrast, a mixture of ceramides, fatty acids, and cholesterol normalized barrier recovery rates. Fluorescent-labeled fatty acids, cholesterol, and ceramides traversed the stratum corneum with uptake into the nucleated layers of the epidermis. Incomplete lipid mixtures produced abnormal lamellar body ultrastructure, leading to abnormal intercellular membrane bilayers and/or phase separation in the intercellular spaces of the stratum corneum. In contrast, lamellar bodies and intercellular structures were normal when complete lipid mixtures were applied. These results suggest that: (1) topical application

18

Concordance of Condylomata Acuminata Responses to Treatment with Intralesional MPI 5003 and Papilloma Responses in the Shope Rabbit Papilloma Model System

John W. Kreider[a], Martin D. Pickel[a], Elaine K. Orenberg[b], Ning Yu[b], Dennis M. Brown[b], Edward Luck[b]
[a] Department of Pathology, The Milton S. Hershey Medical Center, Hershey, Pa., USA; [b] Matrix Pharmaceutical, Inc., Menlo Park, Calif., USA

A new intralesional sustained-release chemotherapy, MPI 5003, is under development as a treatment for condylomata acuminata. MPI 5003 is a biodegradable gel comprised of a protein carrier matrix, tissue modifier (epinephrine) and the drug, 5-fluorouracil (5-FU). This drug product was evaluated in Shope rabbit papillomas to assess responses to a range of intralesional MPI 5003 doses and concordance of responses in the animal model system to drug responses in human condyloma clinical studies. The rabbit papilloma virus (CRPV) has a genome analogous to human papilloma virus. New Zealand white rabbits were inoculated with CRPV viron at two dilutions [10^{-1}, 10^{-2} of a 10% (w/v) extract in saline] at four dorsal sites. After 21 days, papillomas (~ 5 mm in diameter) were injected with MPI 5003 (0.1 ml vol) containing one of 3 doses (0.3, 1.5 or 3.0 mg 5-FU), or placebo, once weekly for 6 weeks. Geometric mean diameters were determined over 10 weeks. MPI 5003 was effective in suppressing growth of Shope papillomas; responses were related to both 5-FU dose and CRPV induction dose. With the lowest MPI 5003 dose (0.3 mg 5-FU), growth inhibition of 43 and 68% was noted in 10^{-1} and 10^{-2} papillomas, respectively. The highest dose (3 mg 5-FU in MPI 5003) inhibited growth of the 10^{-1} papillomas by 75%, and 100% in the 10^{-2} lesions. The 3-mg 5-FU dose that evoked cures in the rabbit papilloma is similar to doses shown to be effective in human condyloma treatments. In phase II clinical studies of 59 patients (103 lesions) treated weekly with MPI 5003 for up to 6 weeks, composite responses show that 90% of treated lesions had ⩾ 50% decrease in wart area, and 75% of the treated lesions had complete responses. The Shope papilloma system was shown to be a useful animal model for study of intralesional chemotherapy with MPI 5003, since lesions were responsive to treatment over a range of drug doses and papilloma virus inoculum. Papilloma responses were in concordance with reductions in condyloma size and complete responses effected by MPI 5003 in human condyloma studies.

19

The Effect of Long-Term Application of 17-Ethylcarbonate-21-Propionate in Symptomatic Dermographism

Susan C. Parker, F. Lawlor, D.M. Francis, R.M. Barr, A. Kobza Black, M.W. Greaves
St. John's Institute of Dermatology, St. Thomas' Hospital, UMDS, London, UK

In symptomatic dermographism (SD) wealing and itching occur after light stroking of the skin. The potent topical steroid clobetasol propionate 0.05% decreases wealing, mast cell numbers and cutaneous histamine levels in SD. 17-Ethylcarbonate-21-propionate (prednicarbate) is a moderately potent corticosteroid which is not absorbed systemically. It may therefore be more suitable for long-term use. We assessed the effect of topical prednicarbate in SD. Prednicarbate and its base were applied double-blind to a 100-cm^2 area on either thigh for 6 weeks with occlusion at night. Transverse weals were produced by the dermographometer at 4 pressures and weal widths were measured at 5 min. At 6 weeks, 4-mm punch biopsies were performed for mast cell counts and histamine assay.

Pascals × 10/mm^2:	Weal width, mm (mean ± SEM, n = 7)			
	2	5.8	9.75	14.12
Prednicarbate	0.0	0.08±0.08	0.51±0.34	0.7±0.42
Base-treated	1.44±0.7	2.01±0.66	3.45±0.53	4.22±0.58

Weal widths were significantly reduced by prednicarbate at the 3 highest pressures (paired t test). Prednicarbate as compared with base-treated sites also decreased mast cell numbers (12.5 ± 5.2 and 27 ± 3.4 cells per 10 HPF, mean ± SEM) and histamine levels (7.8 ± 0.7 and 15 ± 2.3 ng/mg, mean ± SEM). These differences did not reach significance. Although prednicarbate is less effective in reducing mast cell numbers and histamine levels than clobetasol propionate 0.05% [Br J Dermatol 1989; 121: 626], it is effective in reducing wealing in SD.

20

Abnormal Platelet Aggregation in Inflammatory Dermatoses

C. Ivey[a], *N.M. Roberts*[a], *C.P. Page*[b], *R.C.D. Staughton*[a]
[a] Department of Dermatology, Westminster Hospital, and [b] Department of Pharmacology, King's College, London, UK

Platelets have recently been implicated in inflammatory disorders. We have therefore investigated the role of platelets in psoriasis and atopic eczema. In vitro aggregation responses of platelets from patients with psoriasis (severity assessed by PASI score) and eczema (severity assessed by a score incorporating symptoms, signs and area) were compared with those from normal volunteers. Strict criteria were defined to exclude confounding causes of abnormal platelet aggregation. Threshold hyperresponsiveness to thrombin and collagen was observed in patients with psoriasis and eczema, whilst responses to ADP and PAF were within normal limits.

	10^{-7} *M* ADP	0.3 U/ml thrombin	0.15 µg/ml collagen	10^{-12} *M* PAF
Normal (n = 20)	5.5±0.8	5.4±1.4	8.8±1.2	27.9±6.0
Psoriasis (n = 17)	11.8±3.8	17.8±4.1*	25.9±6.0*	50.8±8.5
Eczema (n = 11)	5.6±0.8	12.4±3.1*	14.5±2.1*	40.3±11.0

Mean ± SEM, * $p < 0.05$, Student's t test for unpaired data.

Psoriasis severity [PASI scores of 3.0–36.1 (mean 15.0)] correlated significantly with responsiveness to collagen ($p < 0.05$, Spearman Rank correlation coefficient), whilst eczema severity [ranging from 18 to 81.5 (mean 48.7)] did not correlate with collagen responsiveness ($p = 0.06$). We conclude that platelet aggregation is abnormal in inflammatory dermatoses, and in psoriasis collagen hyperresponsiveness may be a marker of disease severity.

21

Phosphorylation of Tyrosine Residues in the Androgen Receptor Mediates Receptor Activation and Hormone Binding in Human Hair Follicles

Marty E. Sawaya
SUNY Brooklyn Health Science Center, Department of Dermatology, Brooklyn, New York, N.Y., USA

The significance of phosphorylation of the androgen receptor (AR) is becoming more apparent from studies suggesting that specific phosphorylation of tyrosine residues may regulate AR function by altering hormone binding, which then effects AR binding to specific gene sites via a nuclear matrix acceptor protein (NAP). NAP was purified from human hair follicles (HFs) and found to be required for specific binding of the AR to nuclear DNA. The 12-kDa NAP is unique in its specificity for mediating saturable binding of AR when titrated with DNA. Recently, it was found that tyrosine phosphorylation of the AR is important for AR binding to NAP in human HFs. ARs were prepared from the cytosol fractions of human HFs after precipitation with 40% ammonium sulfate. Nuclear ARs were prepared from purified nuclei with micrococcal nuclease and 0.8 *M* NaCl. The effect of phosphatases and phosphatase inhibitors on ^{3}H-dihydrotestosterone (DHT) binding to ARs was examined, as well as AR binding to NAP in the nuclear fractions. The ARs were incubated with a phosphotyrosine monoclonal antibody and an immunoprecipitation protocol was followed. DHT-AR and DHT-AR-NAP binding activity was recovered after immunoprecipitation from nuclear AR fractions, with a recovery of 47% binding activity. Incubation of AR with tetranitromethane and *p*-nitrobenzene sulfonyl fluoride, which modifies tyrosine residues, inhibited steroid binding to the receptor by >95%. These results suggest that specific phosphorylation of tyrosine residues in AR is important in mediating receptor activation and may play an important role in signaling hormone-induced cell growth or inhibitory responses in hair growth.

22

Evaluation of the Potential for Hypothalamic-Pituitary-Adrenal (HPA) Axis Suppression with Halobetasol Propionate Cream, and Ointment Formulations of Halobetasol Propionate, Clobetasol Propionate and Augmented Betamethasone Dipropionate

E.H. Schwarzel[a], *S.B. Siskin*[a], *W.W. Epinette*[a], *J.R. Gibson*[a], *R.A. Blum*[b], *H.I. Katz*[c], *J.C. Kisicki*[d]
[a] Bristol-Meyers Squibb Pharmaceutical Research Institute and [b] Millard Fillmore Hospital, Buffalo, N.Y., USA; [c] Minneapolis Clinical Study Center, Minneapolis, Minn., USA; [d] Harris Laboratories, Lincoln, Nebr., USA

The effect of halobetasol propionate (Ultravate®) on the HPA axis was evaluated in two studies. One study was an open-label trial of halobetasol propionate cream (HC, Ultravate) in 12 subjects and the other was a double-blind, randomized study comparing the ointments halobetasol propionate (HO, Ultravate), clobetasol propionate (CO, Temovate®) and augmented betamethasone dipropionate (BO, Diprolene®) in 36 subjects (12 per group). Medications were applied twice a day for 14 days at the maximum recommended dosage levels (50 g/week for HO, CO, HC and 45 g/week for BO). Plasma and urinary cortisol levels and efficacy evaluations were obtained prior to treatment, during treatment and after treatment. All baseline plasma cortisol levels were within the normal range (5–23 μg/dl). After 7 days of treatment the HO group showed the greatest degree of HPA axis suppression, followed by the CO > HC > BO groups. After 14 days of treatment the order of the four treatment groups was: HC > CO > HO > BO. None of the mean plasma cortisol values after either 7 or 14 days of treatment for any of the treatment groups was below the normal range. During the 14 days of treatment 2 subjects in the HC group, 4 subjects in the HO group, 2 subjects in the CO group and none of the subjects in the BO group had individual plasma cortisol levels below 5 µg/dl. All subjects who had plasma cortisol levels below 5 µg/dl during treatment had values within the normal range at the post-treatment evaluations (4 days after treatment). All subjects showed distinct improvement in their psoriasis during the 14 days of treatment.

It is concluded that halobetasol propionate (Ultravate), in cream and ointment formulations, is an effective super-high potency topical corticosteroid with a safety and efficacy profile typical of this class of compounds.

23

A Short-Term Protocol for Dry Skin Treatments with Physical Measurements of Skin Function

G. Grove[a], *V. Stevens*[b], *J. Gibson*[b]
[a]KGL Skin Study Center, Philadelphia, Pa., USA; [b]Bristol-Myers Squibb Pharmaceutical Research Institute, Buffalo, N.Y., USA

The purpose of this study was to assess an abbreviated, 4.5-day, dry skin protocol to evaluate marketed formulations using clinical grades and physical measurements. This protocol was developed by the KGL Skin Study Center, where the study was conducted. Both 'soap-induced' and 'natural', geriatric dry skin of the lateral lower legs were examined in separate panels of 20 subjects each. After 2 weeks of preconditioning (washout or soap induction), treatment sites were evaluated by clinical grades (9-point scale) and by physical measurements (TEWL, skin conductance, laser-Doppler flowmetry, and dermal torque flexibility). Four lotion formulations, Eucerin®, Lubriderm®, Lac-Hydrin® Five, or placebo were then applied to randomized areas (5 × 10 cm) of the lower leg. These formulations were reapplied twice daily for 4.5 days (9 applications). All physical and clinical evaluations were repeated 6 h after the last application (day 5) and during a regression phase (no treatment) on days 8, 11, and 18. Differences in dry skin grades were observed as early as day 2 of treatment, and statistically significant differences were seen by day 4 and during regression. Lac-Hydrin Five was superior to the other formulations in clinical grades and skin conductance in both the geriatric and soap-induced groups. This difference developed during treatment and continued during the regression phase. These were the most discriminating parameters in this short-term protocol. Evaporimetry was able to identify formulations with occlusive effects during treatment, but the decrease in TEWL was lost during regression. Trends could be observed in the laser-Doppler and dermal torque data, but statistically significant separations in the data from different treatments was not achieved. This short-term protocol should be useful in assessing dry skin products both in treatment and regression phases.

24

Effects of Different Antipsoriatic Therapies on Titers of Antibodies to an Oxidized Thymidine Moiety

D. Khasak[a], *K. Frenkel*[b], *J. Karkoszka*[b], *J. Shupack*[a], *M. Stiller*[a]
[a]Ronald O Perelman Department of Dermatology, and [b]Department of Environmental Medicine, NYU Medical Center, N.Y., USA

Inflammation and exposure to ultraviolet (UV) radiation may result in formation of reactive oxygen species (ROS). Systemic therapy with anti-inflammatory and cytotoxic drugs may decrease ROS. Sera of patients with inflammatory dermatoses contain elevated titers of antibodies (Ab) binding the oxidized thymidine moiety 5-hydroxymethyl-2′-deoxyuridine (HMdU). After determining that anti-HMdU Ab titers were significantly higher in psoriatic patients than in healthy controls (NS, $p < 0.001$), we decided to ascertain the effects of UVB (290–320 nm) phototherapy and of systemic treatment on anti-HMdU Ab titers. Sera of study subjects were analyzed by enzyme-linked immunosorbent assay using microtiter plates coated with HMdU coupled to bovine serum albumin. Psoriatic patients systemically treated with methotrexate and/or oral retinoids had significantly lower anti-HMdU Ab titers (17.4 ± 3.0) than psoriatics not receiving systemic therapy (28.0 ± 4.6) ($p < 0.001$). Levels approached those of NS (15.4 ± 2.0). In contrast, psoriatics receiving UVB phototherapy had significantly higher anti-HMdU Ab titers (42.4 ± 5.1) than other psoriatics ($p < 0.005$). Their titers approached those of patients with cutaneous immune complex diseases (55.4 ± 11.1) not receiving systemic therapy. As with psoriatics, treatment of immune complex diseases with systemic anti-inflammatory and cytotoxic drugs significantly lowered anti-HMdU Ab titers (17.4 ± 3.0, $p < 0.001$). There was no correlation between anti-HMdU Ab titers and erythrocyte sedimentation rates or the presence of C-reactive protein. Assaying anti-HMdU Ab in sera of patients with inflammatory skin disease may be a useful tool in monitoring efficacy of therapy and/or level of disease activity.

25

A Double-Blind, Placebo-Controlled Clinical Trial to Evaluate Thymopentin in the Treatment of Atopic Dermatitis

M.J. Stiller, J.L. Shupack, N.A. Soter
The Ronald O. Perelman Department of
New York University Medical Center, N.Y., USA

Patients with atopic dermatitis (AD), a common chronic inflammatory skin disease, frequently have immunologic abnormalities including defective T-cell function and elevated serum IgE levels. Thymopentin (TP-5), a synthetic pentapeptide corresponding to amino acid residues 32 through 36 of the 48-amino acid immunomodulatory thymic hormone thymopoietin, was evaluated in a double-blind, placebo-controlled clinical trial in patients with severe AD. Thirty-five patients (18 TP-5, 17 placebo) 2 years and older with greater than 20% body surface area AD were randomly assigned to receive either 50 mg of subcutaneous TP-5 thrice weekly or placebo. Patients were permitted to continue oral antihistamines and topical triamcinolone acetonide 0.1% and/or hydrocortisone 1% creams during this 84-day clinical trial. All other therapies for AD were discontinued prior to enrollment. Efficacy parameters included pruritus, erythema, induration (total severity score sum of pruritus, erythema, and induration), lichenification, scaling/dryness, percentage of total body surface area affected, and patient and physician global evaluations. After 84 days, TP-5-treated patients showed a statistically significant improvement compared to their placebo-treated counterparts for erythema ($p = 0.028$), total severity score ($p = 0.055$), lichenification ($p = 0.029$), scaling/dryness ($p = 0.011$), extent of body involvement ($p = 0.001$), and physician global evaluation ($p = 0.006$). No adverse events attributable to TP-5 occurred in our patients. We conclude that TP-5 is a safe, effective alternative therapy for severe AD.

Funded by a grant from Immunobiology Research Institute Annandale, N.J., USA.

26

Cytochrome P4501A1-Dependent Metabolism of Skin Carcinogen Benzo(a)pyrene in Human Langerhans Cells

Jacquelinn A. Studer, Frank K. Jugert, Thomas E. Fleming, Craig A. Elmets, Daniel P. Bik, Rajesh Agarwal, Hasan Mukhtar
Department of Dermatology, University Hospitals of Cleveland, Case Western Reserve University, Cleveland, Ohio, USA

Langerhans cells are antigen-presenting cells in the skin which trigger immune responses. In prior studies we have shown that polycyclic aromatic hydrocarbons such as benzo(a)pyrene and 7,12-dimethylbenz(a)anthracene are able to initiate cell-mediated immune responses. In this study, human Langerhans cells isolated from adult fresh human cadaver skin were incubated in culture medium with [^{3}H]-benzo(a)pyrene at 37 °C for 24 h, and benzo(a)pyrene metabolite formation in sonicated cell lysate and culture medium was assessed by high-pressure liquid chromatography (HPLC). The HPLC analysis indicated the formation of both intracellular and extracellular benzo(a)pyrene metabolites such as phenols, quinones and diols. Significant amounts of [^{3}H]-benzo(a)pyrene metabolites were also identified as glucuronide and sulfate conjugates, both in sonicated cell lysate as well as in medium. Since the first step in the metabolism of benzo(a)pyrene is carried out by the cytochrome P4501A1-dependent enzymatic pathway, we next investigated whether this heme protein is present in human Langerhans cells. The 10,000 *g* supernatant fraction prepared from human Langerhans cells was subjected to sodium dodecyl sulfate-polyacrylamide gel electrophoresis followed by transfer of resolved proteins onto nitrocellulose membrane by Western blotting. Incubation of the membrane with highly specific polyclonal antibody to cytochrome P4501A1 showed an immunoreactive band. Our data indicate that human Langerhans cells possess cytochrome P4501A1, which metabolizes the skin carcinogen benzo(a)pyrene.

27

Inhibition of Protein Kinase C by Antibiotics

Susan M. Toso, Lutz Hegemann, Jouni Uitto, Guy F. Webster
Department of Dermatology, Thomas Jefferson University, Philadelphia, Pa., USA

Tetracyclines are of great importance in the treatment of granulomatous inflammatory diseases of the skin, such as acne and rosacea. We have previously shown that mechanisms of transmembraneous signal transduction involving protein kinase C (PKC) play a key role in the regulation of various pathological responses within the skin, such as inflammation and hyperproliferation. Therefore, we investigated the effects of various antibiotics on the activity of partially purified PKC as well as in an in vitro model of granuloma formation. All antibiotics which are clinically effective in the treatment of granulomatous skin diseases (tetracycline, minocycline, and doxycycline) inhibited the in vitro granuloma formation and PKC activity in a dose-dependent manner, displaying IC_{50} values in the micromolar range. The efficacy of the tetracyclines in the cellular model, with doxycycline being the most potent inhibitor, correlated with the drug's potency to directly inhibit PKC activity in the cell-free assay and reflected their therapeutic activity in clinical use. In contrast, ciprofloxacin, clindamycin, and erythromycin, which are of little therapeutic value in the treatment of granulomatous diseases, inhibited in vitro granuloma formation and PKC activity only marginally. In conclusion, the present data demonstrate that the antigranulomatous drug activity of antibiotics in vivo and in vitro correlates with inhibition of PKC.

28

The Safety of Topically Applied Calcipotriene Ointment 0.005% (a Vitamin D_3 Analogue) as Measured by Blood, Urine and Bone Density Analysis in Psoriatic Patients

R. Wehr[a], J. Gibson[a], W. Epinette[a], S. Pincus[b], C. Chesnut[c], B. Goffe[d], I. Katz[e], C. Guzzo[f], N. Lowe[g]
[a] Bristol-Myers Squibb PRI and [b] State University of New York, Buffalo, N.Y., USA; [c] Northwest Medical Teaching and Research Foundation, [d] Psoriasis Treatment Center, Seattle, Wash., USA; [e] Minnesota Clinical Research, Fridley, Minn., USA; [f] University of Pennsylvania, Philadelphia, Pa., USA; [g] Skin Research Foundation, Santa Monica, Calif., USA

The objective of this study was to evaluate the potential effect of the topical application of the vitamin D_3 analogue calcipotriene on calcium and bone metabolism in psoriatic patients. The active form of vitamin D, 1,25-dihydroxy vitamin D_3, has a profound calcium-mobilizing effect in man when absorbed systemically. An analogue of 1,25-dihydroxy vitamin D_3, calcipotriene, has been shown to have significantly less effect on calcium metabolism while retaining an antiproliferative effect useful in the treatment of psoriasis. This double-blind, parallel-group study of 76 psoriasis patients utilized inpatient hospital clinical research units or designated psoriasis treatment center facilities. Twenty-four-hour urine and fasting blood samples were collected. Dual-energy X-ray absorptiometry or dual-photon absorptiometry were performed within 2 weeks of enrollment and within 2 weeks after drug was stopped. After a washout period, patients were enrolled for an 8-week b.i.d. treatment course. They were evaluated at weeks –2, 0, 1, 2, 4, 6 and 8 for severity of psoriasis in terms of scaling, erythema, plaque elevation, overall lesion severity and a physician's global assessment. A screening blood specimen was taken at week –2 to document serum calcium and other key parameters. Patients were enrolled in the treatment phase of the study at week 0, placed in the inpatient facility and 24-hour urines and fasting blood samples were obtained. This was repeated at weeks 1, 2, 4, and 8. Statistical analysis of the bone density data demonstrated that calcipotriene did not change bone mineral density over the 8-week treatment period. Laboratory data for markers of bone metabolism including urine and serum calcium, urinary hydroxyproline and serum bone-specific alkaline phosphatase showed no significant changes. There was a significant reduction in the severity of psoriasis in the calcipotriene-treated patients compared to the vehicle-treated group. Topical calcipotriene, at doses that significantly reduced psoriasis severity, did not affect calcium metabolism.

29

Photodynamic Therapy of Murine Skin Tumors

S.I.A. Zaidi, R. Agarwal, D.R. Bickers, H. Mukhtar
Department of Dermatology, Case Western Reserve University, University Hospitals of Cleveland, Cleveland, Ohio, USA

Photodynamic therapy (PDT) of cancer is an experimental tumor therapy which relies on the combined use of systemically administered photosensitizer (PS) to a tumor-bearing host and the local illumination of the lesion by high intensity visible light source, typically a tunable argon-dye laser. This results in the ablation of tumor. Until recently, derivatives of hematoporphyrin have been employed for PDT of cancer. Photofrin®-II, a complex mixture of porphyrins, is the only PS currently approved for phase III human clinical trials in the USA. Several laboratories have used Photofrin-based PDT in the management of cutaneous and subcutaneous malignancies in humans. Encouraging results with partial to complete response have been reported. However, because of certain drawbacks, specifically high and extended skin phototoxicity associated with the use of porphyrins, there has been a continued interest in developing new PSs with improved therapeutic efficacy for use in the PDT of cancer. The majority of preclinical data on the efficacy of the PSs in PDT of cancer has been generated using transplanted tumors, which do not originate in their native tissue matrix, a situation that does not mimic human conditions. In this laboratory, Photofrin-II and a series of silicon and aluminum phthalocyanines are being investigated for their PDT responses in tumors induced in murine skin by chemical carcinogens or by ultraviolet B radiation. PDT in animals bearing benign papillomas using 5 mg/kg of Photofrin-II or chloroaluminum phthalocyanine tetrasulfonate (AlPcTS) administered intraperitoneally (i.p.) and irradiated within absorption spectrum of the PS resulted in highly significant to complete tumor ablation. PDT using 1 mg/kg i.p. administered silicon phthalocyanine (SiPc) and dye-laser tuned at 675 nm showed complete tumor necrosis. PDT of murine skin tumors with Photofrin-II showed significant cutaneous photosensitization for at least 6 days after irradiation; AlPcTs and SiPc produced only transient photosensitization. PDT with new improved PSs may be a part of a new armamentarium for the management of human skin tumors especially in patients who are ineligible for conventional therapy.

The 9th SPS Annual Meeting is followed by the meeting announced below. Please note the Joint SDRC/SPS Keynote Lecture and Session.

Skin Diseases Research Center, University Hospitals of Cleveland, Case Western Reserve University, October 16 and 17, 1992, Cleveland, Ohio

In cooperation with the American Cancer Society of Cuyahoga County and the National Institute of Arthritis, Musculoskeletal and Skin Diseases

Environmental Skin Cancer: Mechanisms, Models and Human Relevance

Meeting Program

	Thusday, October 15
17:30	Registration (Ambassador Promenade, Stouffer Lobby)
18:30	Gala Dinner (Crawford Auto Aviation Museum: Meet at Stouffer Lobby to Board Buses)

	Friday, October 16
7:30	**Overview** (Stouffer Ballroom A) David R. Bickers (Cleveland, Ohio)
	Joint SDRC/SPS Keynote Lecture
7:45–8:45	Biochemical and Molecular Changes Relevant to the Pathogenesis of Skin Cancer Stuart Yuspa (Bethesda, Md.)
	Session I (Stouffer Ballroom A) **Mechanisms in Skin Cancer** *Chairman:* Thomas Luger (Munster)
8:45–9:15	Gene Specific DNA Repair: Relevance for Carcinogenic Mechanisms Philip Hanawalt (Stanford, Calif.)
9:15–9:45	Cytochrome P-450 and Environmental Carcinogenesis Frank Gonzalez (Bethesda, Md.)
9:45–10:15	Oxidant Stress and Skin Cancer Peter Cerutti (Lausanne)
10:15–10:45	Coffee Break

	Session II (Stouffer Ballroom A) **Transgenic Mice and Skin Cancer** *Chairman:* Thomas Slaga (Smithville)
10:45–11:15	UV-Induced Melanomas of Transgenic Mice Beatrice Mintz (Philadelphia, Pa.)
11:15–11:45	Transgenic Mouse Models for Skin Cancer Dennis Roop (Houston, Tex.)
	Joint SDRC/SPS Session
11:45–12:45	Albert Kligman Lecture (Stouffer Ballroom A) David Bickers (Cleveland, Ohio)
12:45–14:00	Poster Viewing
	Session III (Ambassador Ballroom) **Viral, Melanoma and UV Cancer** *Chairman:* Kenneth Kraemer (Bethesda, Md.)
14:00–14:30	Models for Melanoma Skin Cancer Ronald Ley (Albuquerque, N. Mex.)
14:30–15:00	Papilloma Virus and Epithelial Cancer Douglas Lowy (Bethesda, Md.)
15:00–15:30	Coffee Break
	Session IV (Ambassador Ballroom) **Immunology and Skin Cancer** *Chairperson:* Margaret Kripke (Houston, Tex.)
15:30–16:00	Cytokines and Malignant Melanoma Thomas Luger (Munster)
16:00–16:30	The Role of Cutaneous Immunity in the Development of Murine and Human Skin Cancers J. Wayne Streilein (Miami, Fla.)
16:30–18:00	Panel Discussion Research Accomplishments and Future Research Needs
18:30	Reception (Oak Room, Tower City Center
20:30	Cleveland Orchestra Concert (Optional)

Saturday, October 17

7:30–8:30	Continental Breakfast (Exhibit Hall)
	Session V (Ambassador Ballroom) **Tumor Promotion and Progression** *Chairman:* Hasan Mukhtar (Cleveland, Ohio)
8:30–9:00	Cellular and Molecular Mechanisms Involved in Skin Tumor Promotion and Progression Thomas Slaga (Smithville)
9:00–9:30	Mechanisms of Skin Tumor Promotion Friedrich Marks (Heidelberg)

9:30–10:00	Roles of Protein Kinase C in Epidermal Growth, Differentiation and Carcinogenesis Toshio Kuroki (Tokyo)
10:00–10:30	Metabolism of Skin Tumor Promoters to Reactive Intermediates Thomas Kensler (Baltimore, Md)
10:30–10:45	Coffee Break

Session VI (Ambassador Ballroom)
Chairman: Friedrich Marks (Heidelberg)

10:45–11:15	Epidemiology of Skin Cancer Joseph Scotto (Bethesda, Md.)
11:15–11:45	Skin Cancer in Maryland Watermen Paul Strickland (Baltimore, Md.)
11:45–12:15	Xeroderma Pigmentosum: Prototype of Environmental-Genetic Interactions in Skin Cancer Kenneth Kraemer (Bethesda, Md.)
12:15–12:45	Chemoprevention of Skin Cancer Hasan Mukhtar (Cleveland, Ohio)

Session VII (Ambassador Ballroom)
Oncogenes/Suppressor Genes
Chairman: Dennis Roop (Houston, Tex.)

14:00–14:30	The Role of Oncogenes and Tumor Suppressor Genes in UV Carcinogenesis H.N. Ananthaswami (Houston, Tex.)
14:30–15:00	The Role of Oncogenes in Skin Cancer Allan Balmain (Glasgow)
15:00–15:30	Tumor Suppressor Gene Mutations in Human Cutaneous Cancer Douglas Brash (New Haven, Conn.)
15:30–16:00	Tumor Suppressor Genes and Skin Cancer Ervin Epstein, Jr. (San Francisco, Calif.)
16:00–17:30	Panel Discussion Research Accomplishments, Future Research Needs
17:30	Closing Remarks David Bickers (Cleveland, Ohio)

Announcement

17th IFSCC in Yokohama

The International Federation of the Society of Cosmetic Chemists will have their 17th International Congress in Yokohama from October 13 through 16 in 1992 just before the 9th ISBN meeting.

For more information, please contact:

Takeo Mitsui, PhD (Chairman, Organizing Committee)
Secretariat
17th IFSCC International Congress Yokohama
c/o Japan Convention Services, Inc.
Nippon Press Center Building 4F
2-2-1 Uchisaiwai-cho, Chiyoda-ku, Tokyo 100 (Japan)
Telephone: (81)–3–3508–1213
Telefax: (81)–3–3508–0820

Sendai International Center
Japan
October 19 and 20, 1992

The International Symposium on Bioengineering and the Skin

Scientific Program

			Abstract No.
		Monday, October 19	
9:30–9:40	**A**	**Opening Remarks**	
9:30		Presidential Address H. Tagami (Sendai)	
9:35		Opening Remarks T. Ozawa (Tokyo)	
9:40–11:30	**B**	**Plenary Session (Room A)**	
9:40–10:00	*PS-I*	*Overview of Bioengineering and the Skin* *Chairpersons:* H.I. Maibach, T. Takeda	
		Bioengineering for Study of the Stratum Corneum – Problems and Solution R. Marks (Cardiff)	
10:00–10:10		Intermission	
10:10–11:30	*PS-II*	*Assessment of Skin Surface* *Chairpersons:* A.M. Kligman, T. Abe	
		Assessment of Skin Irritation with Bioengineering Techniques J. Serup (Copenhagen)	**39**
		Measurement of Skin pH S. Dikstein	
		Skin Surface Contour (I) G.L. Grove (Broomall)	
		Skin Surface Contour (II) M. Takahashi (Yokohama)	
11:30–12:00		Lunch Time	

Note

(1) There might be minor changes of the schedule announced before the symposium.
(2) Since the symposium schedule is very tight, please finish your presentation within the indicated period of time: plenary session: 15 min/person; workshop: 10 min, and concurrent session: 9 min.

Time	Session	Program	Abstract No.
12:00–14:20		***Luncheon Seminar***	
12:00–12:40	*PS-III*	*Skin Hydration* *Chairpersons:* R. Marks, T. Ishida	
		Conductance Measurement H. Tagami (Sendai)	
		Hydration Measurement T. Ozawa (Tokyo)	
12:40–13:00		Intermission	
13:00–13:40	*PS-IV*	*Mechanical and Electrical Properties of the Skin* *Chairpersons:* J.-L. Leveque, Y. Asada	
		Mechanical Measurement of Skin H.G. Vogel (Frankfurt)	**40**
		Measurement and Analysis of Skin Impedance Y. Yamamoto (Okayama)	**41**
13:40–14:20	*PS-V*	*Blood Circulation* *Chairpersons:* J.-L. Leveque, Y. Asada	
		Thermography I. Fujimasa (Tokyo)	**42**
		Cutaneous Blood Flow P.G. Agache (Besançon)	**43**
14:20–15:20	**C**	**Poster and Display Discussion**	**49–61**
15:20–17:10	**D**	**Concurrent Session (Room A)**	
15:20–16:10	*CS-I*	*Mechanical Measurement of the Skin* *Chairpersons:* S. Distein, M. Matsumoto, M. Takahashi	
		An Improved Method for Measurement of Intercorneal Cohesion and Lipids by Tape Stripping Y. Nishimori (Yokohama)	**1**
		Development of a Small Tension Meter System for the Scalp T. Komeda (Saitama)	**2**
		Evaluation of a Skin Stiffness on the Body Surface H. Oka (Okayama)	**3**
16:10–16:20		Intermission	
16:20–17:10	*CS-II*	*Evaluation of Skin Irritation* *Chairpersons:* J. Serup, R. Hayakama, Y. Kuroiwa	
		A New in vitro Technique to Assess the Damaging Effects of Surfactants on Human Stratum Corneum T. Shukuwa (Pennsylvania)	**4**
		Influence of Sweat on Skin Irritancy in a Closed Chamber Y. Ninomiya (Miyagi)	**5**
		A Novel Approach in the Evaluation of Irritancy Potential: The Use of in vivo and in vitro Techniques B. Reece (Dallas)	**6**
17:10–18:50		Intermission	

			Abstract No.
17:20–18:50	**E**	**Workshop I (Room A)** *Chairpersons:* G.L. Grove, K. Hoffmann, K. Okamoto	
	WS-I	*Skin Surface Contour*	
		Profilometry K. Hoffmann (Bochum)	
		Study on an Optical Measuring Method of Skin Aging T. Uchida (Saitama)	**28**
		Optical Profilometry of Replicas – Revisited D.L. Miller (Dallas)	**29**
		The 3-D Shape Representation of Skin Surface Y. Sohmiya (Keio)	**30**
15:20–18:50	**F**	**Concurrent Session (Room B)**	
15:20–16:10	*CS-III*	*Microcirculation* *Chairpersons:* P.G. Agache, I. Fujimasa	
		Patch Test Responses to Rockwool of Different Diameters Evaluated by Cutaneous Blood Flow Measurement H.C. Eun	**7**
		The Effects of Occlusion by PVC Glove Material on the Percutaneous Penetration of Nicotinates in vivo in Subjects with Normal Skin C.J. Graves (Cardiff)	**8**
		Multichannel Laser Doppler Flowmetry with Peltier's Element-Temperature Control Unit M. Kawai (Tokyo)	**9**
16:10–16:20		Intermission	
16:20–17:10	*CS-IV*	*Skin Color* *Chairpersons:* R.R. Anderson, Y. Kuroda	
		Video-Optical Monitoring of the Time-Course of Skin Wheal and Flare Reactions P. Bjerring (Aarhus)	**10**
		Comparison of Skin Color Computer with Dermaspectrometer T. Nakanishi (Osaka)	**11**
		γ-Linoleinic Acid, β-Glycyrrhetinic Acid and Glycerol Triesters and the Suppression of the UVB-Induced Erythema: Evaluation by Reflectance Spectrophotometry M. Silva (Lisbon)	**12**
17:10–17:20		Intermission	
17:20–19:00	*CS-V*	*Skin Hydration and Barrier Function* *Chairpersons:* E. Berardesca, T. Sugai, Y. Morimoto	
		Evaluation by Means of TEWL of the Protective Function of Proteins against Surfactant Aggressivity A. Teglia (Tavernieria)	**13**

			Abstract No.
		Study of the Stratum corneum Barrier Function by Transepidermal Water Loss Measurement: Comparison between Two Commercial Instruments A. Barel (Brussels)	**14**
		Comparison between the Data Obtained with Skin Surface Hygrometer and Those with New Type Tactile Sensor Y. Tanita (Tohoku)	**15**
		Water Sorption-Desorption Behavior in Neonatal Rats: Effects of the Periderm R.R. Wickett (Cincinnati)	**16**
		Irritation as Reflected through Electrical Impedance in Comparison with TEWL, CM, LDF and Visual Scoring S. Ollmar (Huddinge)	**17**
		Moisturizers Influence Barrier Properties of Normal Skin M. Lodén (Stockholm)	**18**
19:30–21:00		**Reception at Shou-Zan-Kan**	

Tuesday, October 20

9:15–10:35	**G**	**Plenary Session (Room A)**	
9:15–10:35	*PS-VI*	*Ultrasound Techniques* *Chairpersons:* R.R. Wickett, Y. Ishibashi	
		Ultrasound Examination of Skin Structures Y. Miki (Ehime)	**44**
		Ultrasound and the Skin: From 5 MHz to the Ultrasound Microscope P. Altmeyer	
		High Frequency Ultrasound of Skin Tumors and Inflammatory Skin Diseases K. Hoffmann (Bochum)	
		Differentiation of the Skin Thinning Potential of Various Topical Glucocorticosteroids by Ultrasound H.C. Korting (Munich)	
10:35–10:45		Intermission	
10:45–11:25	*PS-VII*	*New Bioengineering Techniques (I)* *Chairpersons:* R. Marks, Y. Yamamoto	
		DDS and Transcutaneous Absorption Y. Morimoto (Tokyo)	
		Skin Imaging by NMR J.-L. Leveque	
11:25–12:05	*PS-VIII*	*New Bioengineering Techniques (II)* *Chairpersons:* R. Marks, Y. Yamamoto	
		Optical Spectroscopy in Skin R.R. Anderson (Boston, Mass.)	**45**
		Cutaneous pO_2 and pCO_2 H. Takiwaki (Tokushima)	**46**
12:05–12.35		Lunch Time	

Time	Code	Session / Title	Abstract No.
12:35–13:35		***Luncheon Seminar***	
12:35–13:15	*PS-IX*	*Photoaging and Race* *Chairpersons:* T. Tezuka, K. Toda, H. Shinohara	
		Non-Invasive Methods for Assessing the Structural and Physiologic Changes of Photodamaged Facial Skin A.M. Kligman (Philadelphia)	**47**
		Racial Differences in Skin Function E. Berardesca (Pavia)	**48**
13:15–13:35	*PS-X*	*Past and Future of Bioengineering and the Skin* *Chairpersons:* T. Tezuka, K. Toda, H. Shinohara	
		Bioengineering and the Skin: Legitimate and Illegitimate Science H.I. Maibach (San Francisco, Calif.)	
13:35–14:30	**H**	**Poster and Display Discussion**	**62–74**
14:30–16:10	**I**	**Workshop II (Room A)**	
	WS-II	*Skin Aging and Photoaging* *Chairpersons:* A.M. Kligman, H.G. Vogel	
		Biomechanical Problems from Chronic Photodamage R. Marks (Cardiff)	**31**
		Non-Invasive in vivo Techniques to Differentiate Photodamage and Ageing in Human Skin M. Quan (Cardiff)	**32**
		The Effect of Topical Tretinoin on Photodamaged Skin Surface Parameters A. Sparavigna (Monza)	**33**
		Skin Aging Visualization Using Multi-Media Image Processing System F. Mizoguchi (Tokyo)	**34**
		Quantitation of Skin Texture during the Aging Process by Computer-Based Image Analysis S. Motta (Milan)	**35**
		Discrepancies in Mechanical Measurement of Skin in Assessing Ageing H.G. Vogel (Frankfurt)	**36**
16:10–16:20		Intermission	
16:20–18:00	**J**	**Concurrent Session (Room A)**	
16:20–18:00	*CS-VI*	*New Bioengineering Techniques* *Chairpersons:* R.R. Anderson, H. Takiwaki	
		Quantitative Evaluation of Human Hair Growth by Image Analysis A. Ishino (Shiseido)	**19**
		New 'Human Hand-Like' Tactile Sensor and Its Applications for Bioengineering and the Skin S. Omata (Fukushima)	**20**
		Development of a Stiffness-Meter for the Skin Surface H. Oka (Okayama)	

			Abstract No.
		Quantitative Evaluation of Sebaceous Secretion on the Forehead: Comparison between the Sebumeter and a Microporous Film P. Clarys (Brussels)	**21**
		Two-Dimensional Moisture Measurement of Skin by Infrared Vidicon H. Muraki (Shizuoka)	**22**
		Observation of Skin Moisture of Hairless Mice by Infrared Vidicon A. Date (Shiga)	**23**
14:30–16:10	**K**	**Workshop III (Room B)** *Chairpersons:* S. Seidenari, K. Hoffmann	
14:30–16:10	*WS-III*	*Image Analysis and Other Data Analysis on Ultrasound Recordings*	
		Relevance of Image Analysis J. Serup (Aulnay-sous-Bois)	
		From Qualitative to Quantitative Ultrasound: A Difficult Task B. Querleux	**37**
		Data Reduction and Computerized Analysis of A Scan Ultrasound Signals and Clinical Variables from the Skin C. Edwards (Cardiff)	
		Image Processing on 20 MHz B Scan Recordings S. Seidenari (Modena)	
		Three-Dimensional Computer Reconstruction in High Frequency Ultrasound S. el Gammal (Bochum)	
16:10–18.00	**L**	**Concurrent Session (Room B)** *Chairpersons:* P. Altmeyer, H.C. Korting, K. Ohtsu	
16:10–18:00	*CS-VII*	*Clinical Application of Skin Imaging Techniques*	
		Clinical Application of Ultrasound Techniques K. Hoffmann (Bochum)	
		In vivo Analysis of Water and Lipid Content in Human Skin by High Resolution Magnetic Resonance Imaging B. Querleux	**24**
		Clinical Evaluation of a Magnetic Resonance Imaging for Diagnosing Skin Tumor I. Ono (Fukushima)	**25**
		Comparative Atrophogenicity Potential of Newly Developed Medium Potent Topical Glucocorticosteroids: What High-Frequency Ultrasound Tells Us M.J. Kerscher (Munich)	**26**
		Skin Thickness Measurement Using the SUM A Scan M. Hart (Munich)	**27**
		Age-Dependent Variations of Normal Skin: Image Analysis Processing on 20 MHz B Scan Recordings S. Seidenari (Modena)	**38**
18:00–18:05	**M**	**Closing Remarks (Room A)** Y. Miki (Matsuyama)	

Skin Pharmacol 1992;5:217–244

Sendai International Center
Japan
October 19 and 20, 1992

The International Symposium on Bioengineering and the Skin

Abstracts

Concurrent Session

Mechanical Measurement of the Skin

1

An Improved Method for Measurement of Intercorneal Cohesion and Lipids by Tape Stripping

Y. Nishimori, Y. Suzuki, T. Hata, M. Satoh, H. Nakano
Dermal Research Department, POLA R&D Laboratories, POLA Corporation, Yokohama, Japan

Until now the only procedure of measuring the force of intercorneal cohesion (ICC) has been the cyanoacrylate resin method using a Cohesograph. Recently, we have developed an improved method of measuring the change of ICC and lipids in each layer of stratum corneum by sequential desquamation with adhesive tape.

We used a Cohesograph and silicone-based lipid-free adhesive tape (6 mm in diameter). Analysis of ICC in each layer was possible by measuring stratum corneum samples from the dorsal skin surface of hairless mice. Approximately one layer of stratum corneum was desquamated by each stripping after applying pressure of 100 g/cm^2 on the skin sample. A linear increase of ICC was observed with each successive tape stripping. At the 7th tape stripping, ICC reached its peak and remained constant thereafter (1st: 75.5 g force; 7th: 141.3 g force).

Since the silicone-based adhesive tape is lipid-free, it was possible to examine the composition of lipids extracted from the tape used in each layer. Changes of ICC in hairless mice of various ages and the human forehead of subjects varying between 20 and 70 years of age were observed in this fashion. This improved method will be useful for comparing the qualitative and quantitative change in cohesive factors and the change in ICC in aging and/or damaged skin.

2

Development of a Small Tension Meter System for the Scalp

T. Komeda[a], *T. Uchida*[a], *H. Koyama*[a], *M. Miyagi*[a], *H. Funakubo*[a], *E. Honda*[b], *M. Yanai*[b], *M. Takahashi*[b]
[a] Shibaura Institute of Technology, Saitama, Japan; [b] Shiseido Product Research Laboratories, Kanagawa, Japan

It is said that the scalp tension has a relation with the hair growing; the aim of our study is to clarify this relation. As a first step we developed a small tension meter system to get the scalp tension data in a simple way. The size of this tension meter is 42 mm in diameter, 320 mm in length and the weight is 450 g. It has a load cell to measure the tension, a linear gauge to measure the displacement and the drive mechanism using

1011–0283/92/
0054–0217$2.75/0

a DC motor. For measuring we put the instantaneous adhesive to the tip of the tension meter and attach it to the scalp; then we stretch the scalp using the drive mechanism and get the tension and displacement data every 20 ms by the computer. When the corneum is separated from the scalp, we stop the meaasurement and the stress-strain curve is drawn automatically on the monitor by the computer.

We measured the tension of the different parts of the scalp using this tension meter system and confirmed that the tension of the vertex part of the scalp is higher than that of the temple part; tension between the hair-growing part and the hairless part of the scalp is different.

3

Evaluation of a Skin Stiffness on the Body Surface

H. Oka[a], *T. Yamamoto*[a], *T. Kajikawa*[b], *N. Narahashi*[b]
[a] Fac. Eng., Okayama University, Japan;
[b] Shiseido Inst. Beauty Sciences, Tokyo, Japan

The aim of measurement of the biomechanical properties on body surface includes obtaining an index of skin stiffness and determining the viscoelasticity of body surface. The biomechanical impedance of the human body has three spectra patterns (soft, intermediate and hard pattern). The resonance frequency of impedance gets higher in the order of the soft, intermediate and hard pattern, the tactile sensation to body surface gets harder. The impedance can express the immovability of the skin surface, a kind of skin stiffness, and is much different around 100–300 Hz. Then it is possible to evaluate the skin stiffness with a higher sensitivity, as measuring the biomechanical impedance around these frequencies.

The stiffness meter of the body surface is developed and it made possible a rapid and easy measurement of the skin stiffness. SH is proposed as the new index of skin stiffness and it has the physical meanings in proportion to biomechanical impedance around 250 Hz. Five body areas of a male subject have been measured 3 times each. The largest SH value is obtained on the forehead and the smallest on the thigh; forehead: 43,552, breast: 13,651, on the ribs: 14,620, thigh: 11,646, calf: 13,887. The difference of SH values between the forehead and the thigh is 4 times. On the other hand, the measurement repeatability of the stiffness meter is 2%; then it is considered that we can evaluate the skin stiffness by using the stiffness meter. The palpation can sensitively observe various physical properties with pressuring and moving by hands. An adequate correlation between the SH value and the evaluation by palpation is estimated from the results of measurements by using the silicone gel models.

Evaluation of Skin Irritation

4

A New in vitro Technique to Assess the Damaging Effects of Surfactants on Human Stratum corneum

T. Shukuwa[a], *A.M. Kligman*[a], *M.S. Christensen*[b], *T. Stoudemayer*[b]
[a] Dept. Derm., Univ. Pennsylvania,
[b] Biosearch Lab., Philadelphia, Pa., USA

Surfactants can damage skin in different ways. Impairment of the horny layer barrier is an important event in the development of irritation. We examined the effects of anionic, cationic and nonionic surfactants on isolated sheets of stratum corneum. 8-mm blisters were raised up by suction on the forearms of 8 white and 3 black adult women. After scraping away the viable epidermis, the horny layer was placed in a chamber and exposed to 1% stirred solutions of surfactants at 60 °C. Microliter samples were removed at intervals ranging from 20 to 120 min. The number, size and morphologic changes of corneocytes were evaluated after staining with rhodamine B.

Harsh anionic soaps caused the most damage with a rapid release of corneocytes, accompanied by swelling and morphologic changes of corneocytes culminating in rupture and dissolution of the cells. Non-ionic surfactants were considerably less injurious to the stratum corneum; cationic were generally mild. Black stratum corneum was substantially more resistant to harsh anionic detergents. Minor damage to the horny layer in this model correlates with claims of mildness and with prior experimental studies dealing with swelling and enhanced permeability of isolated horny layers.

5

Influence of Sweat on Skin Irritancy in a Closed Chamber

Collaborative Study of the Third Research Group of Japanese Society for Cutaneous Health

Y. Ninomiya[a], *H. Akita*[b], *J. Kawai*[c], *Y. Kitazawa*[d], *H. Matsumura*[e], *K. Miyata*[f], *T. Mizoguchi*[g], *K. Oka*[h], *M. Okkotsu*[i], *S. Suda*[j], *M. Suzuki*[k], *F. Takazawa*[f], *T. Takei*[l], *K. Tsubota*[m], *K. Kawai*[n, 1], *K. Kawai*[n, 1]
[a]Nitto Denko, Miyagi, Japan; [b]Kyowa, Osaka, Japan; [c]Japanese Society for Cutaneous Health, Kyoto, Japan; [d]Soken Chemical and Engineering, Saitama, Japan; [e]Uni Charm, Shizuoka, Japan; [f]Oji Paper, Tokyo, Japan; [g]Toray Industries, Shiga, Japan; [h]Toyo Chemical, Shiga, Japan; [i]Kanebo-NSC, Osaka, Japan; [j]Nihon Kohden, Tokyo, Japan; [k]Nichiban, Aichi, Japan; [l]Tonen Chemical, Tokyo, Japan; [m]Sekisui Chemical, Medical Research Laboratory, Corporate Research Institute, Osaka, Japan; [n]Kawai Clinic, Kyoto, Japan

The influence of sweat on skin irritancy in a closed chamber was investigated. Closed column shape polyethylene form chambers (∅ 20 × 5 mm), which were tightly covered with several films of different water vapor permeability, were applied on the flexor surface of the upper arms for 24 h. The chamber walls were raised, so that the film did not make direct contact with the skin surface. Thus, only the influence of the humidity in the chambers was evaluated. Skin surface changes were observed under the microscope, using the replica method. There was a negative correlation between the water vapor permeability of the films and skin irritancy. Humidity in the chambers correlated with skin irritancy. The tests were performed 3 times in September, November, and the following February, to investigate the influence of season (i.e. temperature and humidity). There was a tendency for skin irritancy to increase with higher temperatures and higher humidity due to the outer environment.

[1] Not a member of the Third Research Group of Japanese Society for Cutaneous Health.

6

A Novel Approach in the Evaluation of Irritancy Potential: The Use of in vivo and in vitro Techniques

B. Reece, D. Deeds, F. Kohlhepp, M. Rosen
Biophysical Skin Research Laboratory, Mary Kay Cosmetics, Dallas, Tex., USA

Certain chemicals have the ability to either reduce or eliminate some of the observation signs of irritation. Many of these are naturally derived materials isolated from both plants and animals and run the spectrum from complex steroid-like materials to simple amino acids. The mechanisms by which these materials work are largely unknown and have revolved around three main schools of thought: (1) complexation with the irritant(s), (2) preventing contact of the irritant with the skin, and (3) the blocking of reaction sites on the skin. The purpose of this paper is 2-fold: (1) evaluate the in vivo ability of two materials to diminish the effects of a known dermal irritant, sodium lauryl sulfate, using biophysical techniques and (2) evaluate the in vitro effects of these chemicals on two inflammatory mediators.

Microcirculation

7

Patch Test Responses to Rockwool of Different Diameters Evaluated by Cutaneous Blood Flow Measurement

Hee Chul Eun[a], *Ho Gyun Lee*[a], *Nam Won Pail*[b]
[a]Department of Dermatology, College of Medicine, Seoul National University and [b]Division of Industrial Health, School of Public Health, Seoul National University, Korea

Rockwool is a man-made mineral fiber used mainly for insulation, which can cause mechanical skin irritation. This study was performed to evaluate the irritant potential of rockwools of different diameters and compare the change of blood flow, measured by laser Doppler flowmetry, at different occlusion times with rockwool. Rockwool A (mean diameter 4.20 ± 1.96 μm) was more irritating than rockwool B (mean diameter 3.20 ± 1.5 μm). The difference was more clearly observed in a 48-hour patch test than in an 8- or 24-hour test. We concluded that the laser Doppler blood flow measurement was a useful experimental tool for the evaluation of irritant patch test response to mechanical irritants like rockwool, and that the 48-hour or more of occlusion time was necessary for certain types of rockwool.

8

The Effects of Occlusion by PVC Glove Material on the Percutaneous Penetration of Nicotinates in vivo in Subjects with Normal Skin

C.J. Graves, C. Edwards, R. Marks
University of Wales College of Medicine, Cardiff, UK

The protection offered by gloves is usually occlusive by nature. This may be counterproductive, as it may alter the stratum corneum and reduce the protective barrier properties of the skin. We are interested in measuring any change in percorneal permeability, after occlusion of the skin by PVC glove material. A relatively simple method [1], using time to onset of topical nicotinate-induced hyperaemia, would seem to offer a good estimate of stratum corneum permeability within clearly defined restrictions. Measurements are made using a laser Doppler flowmeter. All blood flow measurements were taken from an experimentally challenged site and from a closely adjacent 'normal' site, and the results expressed as either differences or ratios of these two sites. In this way differences in physiological reaction to the nicotinate between subjects were controlled for.

Changes in percorneal permeability were measured after occlusion of the forearm skin of 10 subjects using 3 × 5 cm patches of PVC glove material. This was done by measuring the change in time to onset of hyperaemia after application of topical hexyl nicotinate. After 4 h occlusion there was a median reduction in the time to onset of hyperaemia, to 59% of its pre-occlusion value (95% confidence interval 41–76%, p = 0.006 Wilcoxon test). After 8 h occlusion this was further reduced to 38% of its pre-occlusion value (95% confidence interval 22–53%, p = 0.006 Wilcoxon test). However onset times returned to normal after an overnight rest period. This indicates that percorneal permeability is increased by the use of occlusive glove material, albeit only temporarily.

9

Multichannel Laser Doppler Flowmetry with Peltier's Element-Temperature Control Unit

M. Kawai, Y. Nagashima, K. Matsuo, A. Akazaki, T. Kamiya, M. Hattori, G. Imokawa
Kao Laboratories, Tokyo, and Tochigi, Japan

In an effort to analyze physiological responses of face skin to temperature, we have devised multichannel laser Doppler flow-metry combined with Peltier's element temperature control unit in which blood flow within tissue and skin surface temperature can be measured simultaneously. Analysis of healthy females (15–59 years, n = 63) demonstrated that the blood flow is well correlated by skin temperature in the cheek but not in the forearm. When the cheek temperatures were decreased by decreasing temperatures with Peltier's element, temperature-induced changes of blood flow showed the following three typical pattners: (1) blood flow increases with decreasing temperature as seen in subjects with both an advance lower blood flow and skin temperature, (2) it is steady at the same level and skin temperature decreases markedly as seen in subjects with an advance moderate blood flow, and (3) it decreases but skin temperature scarcely decreases as seen in aged subjects with both an advance higher blood flow and skin temperature. These cutaneous sensitivities to temperature will be discussed in relation to the corresponding skin conditions.

Skin Color

10

Video-Optical Monitoring of the Time Course of Skin Wheal and Flare Reactions

P. Bjerring[a], J. Lauridsen[b], L. Arendt-Nielsen[b]
[a] Department of Dermatology, University Hospital of Aarhus, Denmark; [b] Department of Medical Informatics, University of Aalborg, Denmark

Monitoring of acute skin inflammatory reactions after intradermal application of different inflammatory mediators can be performed by measurement of the cutaneous wheal and flare reaction. Previously, these reactions have been measured by either tracing the circumference of the visually determined areas by a pen on a plastic sheet for subsequent planimetric determinations of areas or by the mean of measurement of two orthogonal diameters of the reactions. However, these methods are subjective measures, and the quality of the test depends on the skill of the investigator. In the case of measurement of flare reactions, manipulation of the skin during measurement may even influence the flare reaction areas. We developed a nontouching procedure, using a video camera for registration of the wheal and flare reactions. The method is based on digital subtraction of pictures, performed after computerized alignment of control and test pictures. Wheal and flare area measurements can be performed with regular intervals, e.g. every minute to obtain information on the dynamics of inflammatory reactions. The time course of the wheal and flare reactions may be of interest especially for determining the physiological target of newly identified inflammatory mediators, e.g. interleukines. Also, the method is suited for determining and comparing the anti-inflammatory action of different topical and systemically administered drugs on standardized acute experimental skin inflammation.

11

Comparison of Skin Color Computer with Dermaspectrometer

T. Nakanishi, T. Sugai
Department of Dermatology, Osaka Kaisei Hospital, Japan

The tristimulus values of colors which portwine stain nevus, nevus spilus and blue nevus revealed were previously reported in Munsell values automatically converted with a skin color computer made by the Pola Laboratories. The apparatus is composed of a tungsten lump, 4 filters and 4 photoelectric circuits. Actual assay of the color is expressed as tristimulus values, X, Y and Z, converted to L*, a* and b*, and then to approximate Munsell values, lightness, chroma and hue, in a computer system. Red color of portwine stain showed a significantly higher value in hue than colors of the other two nevi ($\alpha = 0.01$). Blue color of blue nevus showed a significantly higher value in chroma than the other two nevi ($\alpha = 0.01$), and also brown color of nevus spilus revealed a significantly higher value in chroma than red color of portwine stain ($\alpha = 0.05$). No significant difference was found in lightness among the three nevi.

On the contrary, dermaspectrometer emits green and red light, measuring the absorption coefficients in the skin, and reads out the erythema/melanin index. It is simple and available for practical use, but impossible to express an actual color.

12

γ-Linolenic Acid, β-Glycyrrhetinic Acid and Glycerol Triesters and the Suppression of the UVB-Induced Erythema: Evaluation by Reflectance Spectrophotometry

M.R. Silva, A.M. Nunes, R.T. Bello, A.P. Soares
Department of Dermatology, Hospital do Desterro, Lisbon, Portugal

By using an experimental model of UVB-induced inflammation, the authors studied by means of reflectance spectrophotometry the suppressive effect on erythema of different topics, which included γ-linolenic acid, β-glycyrrhetinic acid, glycerol triesters, indomethacin and hydrocortisone. The results are discussed on the basis of the physiopathological mechanism of the UVB radiation-induced erythema.

Skin Hydration and Barrier Function

13

Evaluation by Means of TEWL of the Protective Function of Proteins against Surfactant Aggressivity

A. Teglia[a], G. Secchi[b]
[a]Kelisema, Taverneria, Italy; [b]G.F. Secchi, Erba, Italy

Animal and vegetable protein hydrolysates with different molecular characteristics were taken from the market or especially prepared for the test and evaluated and compared relative to their reduction potential of sodium lauryl sulfate irritancy. After application of occlusive skin chamber, the transepidermal water loss (TEWL) was tested using a new instrument based on the law of diffusion (A. Fick), measuring the quantity of water evaporated by the skin surface. Contemporaneously visual scoring of skin irritation and moisture content measurements of the horny layer with electric capacitance method were made.

14

Study of the Stratum corneum Barrier Function by Transepidermal Water Loss Measurements: Comparison between Two commercial Instruments (Evaporimeter® and Tewameter®)

A. Barel, P. Clarys
Algemene en Biologische Scheikunde, Vrije Universiteit Brussel, Belgium

The measurement of Transepidermal Water Loss (TEWL) is an important noninvasive method in order to assess the barrier function of the stratum corneum.

As a consequence, TEWL has been found to be a very useful technique for studying skin irritation induced by various physical and chemical effects. Exposure of the skin to chemicals (irritants) and physical conditions (occlusion and stripping) generally results in an increase of TEWL.

Until now the only commercially available TEWL instrument was the Evaporimeter®, developed by Servo Med (Sweden). The open chamber measuring system is based on 2 humidity and temperature sensors which measure the water evaporation gradient at the surface of the skin. Recently a new commercially available instrument, based on the same principle of measurement was developed by Courage and Khazaka (Tewameter®, FRG).

Our aim in this study was to compare the measuring capacities of both instruments. The accuracy, sensitivity, variability, reproducibility and convenience of use of both instruments were compared on normal skin and skin damaged by external factors. Finally the 2 instruments were compared in practice when following the increase of TEWL resulting from exposure of the hands and the forearms to different irritants (detergents and a bleaching product).

15

Comparison between the data obtained with Skin Surface Hygrometer and Those with New-Type Tactile Sensor

Yasuo Tanita[a], *Katuko Kikuchi*[a], *Hachiro Tagami*[a], *Osamu Osanai*[b], *Shuichi Akasaki*[b], *Michio Kawai*[b], *Genji Imokawa*[b], *Sadao Omata*[c]
[a]Tohoku University, Japan; [b]Kao Research Laboratories, Japan; [c]College of Engineering, Nihon University, Japan

Until now, mechanical properties of the skin have been measured by applying various forces such as traction, tension, elevation, indentation, suction, and vibration; although each method has its merits and demerits, there are still no satisfactory methods.

Using a new type of tactile sensor designed to detect a shift in resonant frequency generated in the piezoelectric element, we measured the skin and compared the data with those obtained with the skin surface hygrometer.

We demonstrate the results revealing that instruments yield data closely related to the skin surface hydration state.

16

Water Sorption-Desorption Behavior in Neonatal Rats: Effects of the Periderma

R. Randall Wickett[a], *J. Mutschelknaus*[a], *S.B. Hoath*[b]
[a]College of Pharmacy and [b]Children's Hospital Medical Center, University of Cincinnati, Ohio, USA

Ontogeny of water sorption-desorption behavior in neonatal rat skin in vivo was investigated using a capacitance technique to monitor relative water content. Exposure of the skin surface to water leads to increased capacitance, which decreases as the skin dries. In full-term newborn rats water sorption appears to be limited and desorption is very rapid. Skin temperature also returns to baseline levels very rapidly. By day 3 after birth water sorption-desorption profiles are characteristic of older animals or adult humans. Growth-retarded animals develop increased water sorption more slowly and growth-enhanced animals develop it more rapidly. A single tape stripping on the day of birth (day 0) leads immediately to sorption-desorption curves virtually identical to those that develop by day 3 in unstripped animals. Microscope of alkaline expanded stratum corneum shows that this single striping removes only the periderm leaving the stratum corneum essentially intact. We interpret these results to indicate that the periderm is a hydrophobic layer with an adaptive thermoregulatory function in newborn rats.

17

Irritation as Reflected through Electrical Impedance in Comparison with TEWL, CM, LDF and Visual Scoring

S. Ollmar[a], *M. Nyrén*[b], *I. Nicander*[a], *L. Emtestam*[b]
[a] Karolinska Institute and [b] Huddinge University Hospital, Department of Dermatology, Huddinge, Sweden

During the last 70 years most human tissue types, including skin, have been investigated regarding their electrical properties. Prior noninvasive impedance techniques have suffered from a lack of discrimination between the different layers of the skin, thus including artifacts from layers without interest in a particular diagnostic situation. We have used a new device which makes possible local measurements of impedance to a controlled depth, and compared it with results obtained with other noninvasive techniques.

Sodium lauryl sulphate with concentrations in the range 0.1–5.0% plus blank was applied in Finn chambers on the volar forearm of healthy volunteers. Exposure time was 24 h. Reading was done before application, and 1 h, 24 h, 1 week and 2 weeks after removal. Thus, both the degree of damage and the healing process were monitored.

At the highest concentration, all methods except the Corneometer exhibited maximum response immediately after removal of patches. The Corneometer exhibited maximum response after about 1 week, and thus appears to reflect the healing process only. Laser Doppler flowmetry was affected by fluctuations difficult to control, and the level of significance was thus hampered. A good agreement between impedance, transepidermic water loss and visual readings was found. An earlier study has shown impedance to correlate with SLS concentrations well below the detection limit of visual readings.

18

Moisturizers Influence Barrier Properties of Normal Skin

M. Lodén[a, b], *M. Lindberg*[b]
[a] ACO HUD, Stockholm, Sweden; [b] Department of Dermatology, University Hospital, Uppsala, Sweden

Biophysical measurements were used to study the influence of moisturizers on the barrier function. The moisturizers were used on the volar forearm twice daily for 20 days. The skin was cleaned well in advance prior to the measurements.

The degree of hydration seems to increase by the regular use of the moisturizers, as indicated by the significant increase in the capacitance measured with a Corneometer CM 820. One of the moisturizers lowered the transepidermal water loss, TEWL, whereas the other did not influence the barrier function. The improved barrier function was verified by exposure of the skin to an irritant. The reaction on the treated area was significantly lower than on the untreated skin.

The results indicate that moisturizers could render normal skin less susceptible to irritants and allergens in the environment.

New Bioengineering Techniques

19

Quantitative Evaluation of Human Hair Growth by Image Analysis

A. Ishino[a], *S. Takahashi*[b], *M. Uzuka*[a], *Y. Morikawa*[a]
[a] Skin Biology Research Lab, Shiseido Research Center, Yokohama, Japan; [b] R&D Plannig Division, Shiseido, Tokyo, Japan

Several methods for quantitative evaluation of human hair growth have been reported. A phototrichogram is a standard technique to obtain an anagen/telogen ratio. Some investigators have attempted to obtain this ratio with a computer-assisted image analysis. However, the quantitation by the image analysis encountered such difficulties as (1) obtaining the same site over repeated examinations, (2) setting up a binary threshold level, which was related to the distinction between hair and background, (3) identifying each individual hair and (4) disposing of overlapping hairs.

We have now improved the image analysis system and developed a software in order to overcome these problems. In this study, the anagen/telogen ratio measured by our new system is compared with a standard phototrichogram method. Results indicate that our new image analysis method can effectively evaluate the anagen/telogen ratio, and further provides additional parameters such as hair size and hair growth rates.

20

New 'Human-Hand-Like' Tactile Sensor and Its Applications for Bioengineering and the Skin

S. Omata
College of Engineering, Nihon University, Tokusada Koriyama Fukushima, Japan

In general, a medical examination by human touch is very important for exploring the shape and texture of a tumor, and it is excellent for detecting the physical properties of living tissue. However, such palpation is frequently performed by the doctor, but it is difficult to detect clearly the difference in the stiffness of skin.

Thus we have developed the new type of tactile sensor which is designed to operate with a piezoelectric element. The sensor, which is 20 mm in length and 1 mm in thickness, is able to detect – very much like the human hand – the hardness and/or softness of an object. Several experiments have been carried out to investigate its possibility of applications for bioengineering and the skin.

The experimental results obtained here indicate that the skin elasticity depends on sex and age: in general, the skin elasticity of a female's cheek is lower than a male's cheek. These levels continue to decrease for a female until her mid-20s when they remain constant. Furthermore, it has been demonstrated with the newly developed procedure that the skin before massaging the male's and female's cheek appears to be elastic, but after massaging the cheek it becomes soft and plastic.

Consequently, since the new sensor is capable of clearly sensing differences in hardness and/or softness of living tissue, it will be used in the field of medicine and cosmetic.

21

Quantitative Evaluation of Sebaceous Secretion on the Forehead: Comparison between the Sebumeter® and a Microporous Film (Sebutape®)

P. Clarys, L. Dhaenens, A. Barel
Algemene en Biologische Scheikunde, Vrije Universiteit Brussel, Belgium

Various noninvasive methods have been developed in order to quantify the amount of skin surface lipids for dermatological and cosmetic purposes. In this study we compare the photometric method of the Sebumeter (increase of light transmission of a plastic film which has absorbed sebum) and the Sebutape (hydrophobic porous film). Sebum excretion rates and causal levels were computed from measurements with the Sebumeter. After removal of the Sebutape from the skin, the tape was sealed on a black surface and quantitative analysis of the total surface of the black spots was performed by image analysis in order to obtain data on sebum excretion rate. Measurements were carried out on the foreheads of different groups of volunteers under standardized experimental conditions. The influence of age, sex and hormonal status in the case of women was evaluated. Good agreement was found between the measurements of sebum excretion rate by the two experimental methods.

22

Two-Dimensional Moisture Measurement of Skin by Infrared Vidicon

H. Muraki[a], *H. Satou*[a], *K. Okumura*[a], *M. Hiramatsu*[a], *A. Date*[b], *T. Yoshii*[b]
[a] Hamamatsu Photonics K.K. Hamakita, Shizuoka, Japan; [b] Procter & Gamble Far East, Yasu, Shiga, Japan

Water molecules strongly absorb near infrared light. Therefore, it is possible to measure moisture content in skin two-dimensionally by an infrared sensitive TV camera (infrared vidicon).

Our measurement system is composed of an infrared vidicon as an image detector, an optical system collecting diffuse reflected light from a sample, an optical interference filter allowing to pass light at desired wavelengths, a tungsten lamp as a light source, and an image processor. This system enables us to collect diffuse reflected infrared images at several wavelengths (1.45, 1.68, 1.80 and 1.94 μm) and also to apply arithmetic operations to the images. The transmission measurement of sliced samples (guinea pig) by a spectrophotometer with an integrating sphere revealed that the penetration depths through the skin at 1.45, 1.68, 1.80, and 1.94 μm are 0.3, 2, 0.5, and 0.2 mm, respectively. Therefore, the image at each wavelength is derived from the absorption by water lying within the corresponding penetration depth. To begin with, we applied this method to the model of in vivo stratum corneum presented by Tagami et al. We confirmed that the infrared imaging method reflects the amount of moisture in stratum corneum, as the conductance measurement does.

The two-dimensional measurement system employing an infrared vidicon proved to be effective to measure moisture content in skin two-dimensionally.

23

Observation of Skin Moisture of Hairless Mice by Infrared Vidicon

A. Date[a], *T. Yoshii*[a], *H. Muraki*[b], *H. Satou*[b], *K. Okumura*[b], *M. Hiramatsu*[b]
[a]Procter & Gamble Far East, Yasu, Shiga, Japan;
[b]Hamatsu Photonics, K.K., Shizuoka, Japan

The two-dimensional moisture measurement system we developed has been proved to be effective to measure skin moisture by using models of stratum corneum sheets and sliced skin. It was found that the moisture images obtained by infrared vidicon were related closely to the skin moisture at internal layers as well as at skin surface. Based on the results, noninvasive moisture measurements were conducted on differently aged hairless mice by using infrared vidicon and skin surface hydrometer. The moisture images by infrared vidicon changed by age, while the conductance by skin surface hydrometer did not change by age. The results of the above two instrumental methods showed that the moisture of living skin including internal layer changed with aging more than that of skin surface.

Clinical Application of Skin Imaging Techniques

24

In vivo Analysis of Water and Lipid Content in Human Skin by High Resolution Magnetic Resonance Imaging

B. Querleux[a], *S. Richard*[a], *J. Bittoun*[b], *O. Jolivet*[b], *I. Idy-Peretti*[b], *R. Bazin*[a], *J.L. Leveque*[a]
[a]Laboratoires de Recherche de L'Oréal, France;
[b]Centre Inter-Etablissement de Résonance Magnétique (CIERM), Hôpital de Bicêtre, France

Introduction. Magnetic resonance imaging (MRI) is a powerful noninvasive method allowing quantitation of proton density in tissues. In this paper we present 2 methods which analyze the water behavior and the water/lipids ratio in the different skin layers.

Materials and Methods. Material: High resolution MR images of the skin in vivo were obtained by connecting to a whole-body 1.5-tesla imager a specific surface gradient coil in the anteroposterior direction in order to achieve an in-depth resolution of about 70 μm, and a small surface RF coil, used in reception, in order to improve the signal to noise ratio. Acquisition Protocols: (1) From the measurement of T1 and T2 values of the skin layers, it is possible to calculate a density of mobile protons per volume unit in each layer. The percentage of the fixed protons fraction can be deduced from the a priori knowledge of the water content of the tissue. (2) By using a 'Dixon 3 points' imaging sequence which consists of the acquisition of 3 MR images corresponding to 3 temporal shifts (t, 0 and −t), we obtain after data processing an image representing only water content and another image representing only lipid content of the tissues.

Results. These 2 quantitative methods characterizing the skin layers will be illustrated by numerous MR skin images obtained on different parts of the body. For example, hydration profiles of stratum corneum in heel under treatment will be presented.

Conclusion. High resolution MRI of the skin in vivo establishes an attractive noninvasive method for the study of the physicochemical properties of the different skin layers.

25

Clinical Evaluation of a Magnetic Resonance Imaging for Diagnosing Skin Tumors

I. Ono, F. Kaneko, N. Gunji, K. Suda, H. Harada
Department of Dermatology, Fukushima Medical College, Japan

For the appropriate surgical treatment of malignant tumors, it is important to clarify the depth and area of invasion of tumors and the relation to surrounding normal tissues such as adipose tissue, muscles and bones in addition to the histological diagnosis of the tumors before the operation. For this purpose we clinically evaluated a magnetic resonance imaging (MRI) for diagnosing skin tumors. A MRI, SIGNA (GE), was used and the analysis was carried out in a spin echo method (TR 1500, TE 20) in this study, and 29 slices of MRI images were accumulated crossing those tumors. The usefulness of a three-dimensional presentation of skin tumors performed by the MRI data was also discussed. For the three-dimensional presentation, Voxelflinger™ was applied and these images were compared with a cross-section of those tumors during operation and histological specimens. We applied the MRI examination on patients with malignant melanoma, malignant fibrous histiocytoma, fibrosarcoma and squamous cell carcinoma of the skin.

MRI was a very useful tool to clarify the depth and area of invasion of malignant tumors and the relation to surrounding normal tissues. MRI is most remarkable when applied to patients with malignant melanoma of soles. A three-dimensional presentation obtained from the MRI data is also useful to understand the three-dimensional condition of those tumors but it still seems to have limitations because of the analytical software of the computer.

26

Comparative Atrophogenicity Potential of Newly Developed Medium Potent Topical Glucocorticoids: What High Frequency Ultrasound Tells Us

M.J. Kerscher, H. Hart, H.C. Korting
Department of Dermatology,
Ludwig-Maximilians-Universität, Munich, FRG

Topical glucocorticoids still belong to the drugs most often used in dermatology. Their use today is limited by the fear of unwanted side effects, in particular skin atrophy. Therefore, several attempts have been made to develop new glucocorticoids showing fewer unwanted side effects. With the advent of mometasone furoate, a newly formulated chlorinated synthetic heterocyclic glucocorticoid, as well as with nonhalogenated double esters such as prednicarbate this problem might be solved.

In a comparative double-blind randomized trial using the DUB 20 ultrasound imaging system 24 healthy volunteers applied two out of the four following preparations once or twice daily: mometasone furoate once daily, the corresponding vehicle, prednicarbate ointment, hydrocortisone 1% ointment, each of them twice daily. Skin thickness was determined on days 0, 4, 7, 14, 21, 28, 35, 42 and 63 by a 20-MHz ultrasound imaging system (DUB 20) using A and B scans.

The results obtained imply that topical glucocorticoids of different types clinically superior to hydrocortisone can be considered safe in terms of skin atrophy. It appears particularly interesting that this does not only apply to glucocorticoids efficacious for eczema but also for congeners used in psoriasis.

In conclusion, our findings imply an increased therapeutic index with some newly developed topical glucocorticoids.

27

Skin Thickness Measurement Using the Sum A Scan

H. Hart, M.J. Kerscher, H.C. Korting
Department of Dermatology, LMU, Munich, FRG

Ultrasound imaging systems of the skin have been available for about 10 years, and skin thickness measurement is now well established. We use the DUB 20 system (tpm, Lüneburg, FRG) which makes A and B scan imaging possible with a special 20-MHz transducer. Thereby, the motor-controlled applicator registers and assembles ultrasound signals into a sectional image of 12.8 mm length. This B mode image is displayed after computer storing and processing of 128 A scans. Up to now, skin thickness was determined on the basis of 5 representative A scans being superimposed on a B scan. Exact measurements, however, often were difficult because of isles of subcutaneous tissue and blood vessels on the border between cutis and subcutis. Conventional A scan imaging often showed two or more amplitude peaks. This problem has been solved by new software of tpm which has introduced the measurement based on a sum A scan. Thus, the microcomputer averages all 128 A scans so that there is always just one exact amplitude peak on the border between cutis and subcutis. Quick and reproducible measurements are feasible.

The advantage of this new method has turned out in a double-blind randomized trial to evaluate the atrophogenicity potential of the following different treatment modalities: mometasone furoate ointment, the corresponding vehicle, prednicarbate ointment and hydrocortisone 1% ointment.

In particular, the increase in reproducibility deserves interest facing the nowadays generally adapted good clinical practice procedures for drug trials.

Workshop

Skin Surface Contour

28

Study on an Optical Measuring Method of Skin Aging

T. Uchida[a], *T. Komeda*[a], *H. Koyama*[a], *M. Miyagi*[a], *H. Funakubo*[a], *K. Harii*[b], *K. Oshima*[c], *Y. Yamaguchi*[d]

[a] Shibaura Institute of Technology, Saitama, Japan; [b] Fac. Medicine, Univ. Tokyo, Japan; [c] Akitsu Inst. Severely Handicapped, Tokyo, Japan; [d] Mitsutoyo, Kanagawa, Japan

Our study aims at finding a quantitative relation between skin aging and a skin surface contour by measuring a surface contour of a negative replica of skin with a three-dimensional optical measuring system. The optical measuring system consists of a laser measuring instrument, an X-Y sliding table, and a personal computer. The laser measuring instrument allows us to measure the distance between the sensor in the measuring instrument and the surface of the replica. Therefore we can carry out three-dimensional measurements of a skin surface contour by scanning the surface of the negative replica two-dimensionally with the X-Y sliding table.

We measured skin surface contours of the back of the hand of male subjects from young to aged. The results of measurements showed that skin surface contours of the young age group had a clear pattern of ridges and grooves while those of the old age group lost the clear pattern with age. Therefore we concluded that the pattern of ridges and grooves on a skin surface had a close relationship to aging. In order to obtain the quantitative index of aging, we also conducted spatial frequency analysis of measured data of skin surface contours by two-dimensional Fourier Transform. From the results of frequency analysis, we found that skin surface contours of the young age group showed the special feature in high spatial frequency compared with those of the old age group.

29

Optical Profilometry of Replicas – Revisited

D.L. Miller

bioNET, Dallas, Tex., USA

In this poster we examine an alternative lighting scheme for rendering skin surface replicas. The common use of highly unidirectional lighting for examining replicas for shadow detail (i.e. wrinkle characterization) is sensitive to operator bias. Furthermore the gray level histogram has no direct relationship to height variation. We propose using an extended, diffuse circular light source that completely surrounds the replica and is in approximately the same plane as the replica surface. Under these conditions, the luminance of the surface when viewed from above faithfully renders the local elevation of the replica surface regardless of orientation. The differences between the two approaches and their advantages and disadvantages are discussed and illustrated.

30
The 3-D Shape Representation of Skin Surface

Y. Sohmiya[a], *S. Ozawa*[a], *M. Takahashi*[b], *Y. Kawajiri*[b]
[a] Keio University;
[b] Shiseido Research Center, Japan

We reported a simple and direct quantitative method [1] which can analyze the microtopographic feature of skin surface using image processing (Shiseido beauty processor). It gives us such characteristic skin parameters as the orientation of ridges and furrows, the size and number of pores, and the degree of skin surface relief through a gray scale image and binarized one. We now wish to report further improvement to this instrument, which is the method of 3-D shape representation of skin surface from gray scale image by a photometric stereo technique.

Usually, many light sources or slit light sources are required to get 3-D information. We have reconstructed 3-D skin profile using only three light sources systems with the application of a flat surface model and the least square error method. With this method the gray scale image of skin surface is devided into many small regions and then, the coefficients of flat surface equation in each region are estimated. We will show some results of a 3-D image obtained from skin surface replica using photometric technique.

1 Y. Nakayama et al.: Cosmet Dermatol 1986;1:187–196.

Skin Aging and Photoaging

31
Biomechanical Problems from Chronic Photodamage

R. Marks, C. Edwards, A. Anstey
Department of Dermatology, University of Wales College of Medicine, Heath Park, Cardiff, UK

Photodamaged skin shows a constellation of physical signs due to alteration in skin structure. Most of the changes are due to changes in the dermal connective tissue and result in physical signs such as wrinkling, alteration in skin colour and telangiectasia.

This paper will review data on the altered mechanical properties of sun-damaged skin and will offer explanations for the physical signs noted. New data using both extensometry and a novel device known as the turgometer will be presented, as will data on skin colour and blood flow. It is suggested that a major determinant of the altered appearance of photodamaged skin is the result of failure of mechanical support to the dermal vasculature.

32
Non-Invasive in vivo Techniques to Differentiate Photodamage and Ageing in Human Skin

M.B. Quan, C. Edwards, R. Marks
Department of Dermatology, University of Wales College of Medicine, Cardiff, UK

Differentiating between the processes of chronological ageing and photodamage in skin is difficult because most people with clinical signs of sun damage are elderly and have experienced both processes.

We have used non-invasive measurements of thickness, elasticity and roughness to assess sites of differing sun exposure in groups of young and older subjects. A young group (age 20–28 years, $n = 6$) and an older group (age 54–79 years, $n = 16$) of white males of phototypes, 1, 2 or 3 were assessed... The extensor forearm, the flexor forearm and the lateral thigh were examined (sites 1, 2 and 3). Skin on site 1 was thicker in the older group ($p = 0.035$), but this was reversed on the other sites. This suggests that thickening from sun damage was greater than thinning due to age on this site of maximum exposure. Replica profilometry showed that roughness parameters (R_a, R_z) were significantly positively correlated with age (R_a: $p = 0.02$; R_z: $p = 0.03$), and negatively but not significantly correlated with histological assessments of photodamage.

Elasticity measurements showed that at all sites the older group had longer relaxation time constants (τ). This could be due to age or increased sun exposure. However, on the most exposed site τ correlated with the histological assessment of photodamage, and statistical analyses showed no relationship between elasticity parameters and age for our volunteers.

These results suggest that skin roughness parameters are strong indicators of age while elasticity measurements are fair predictors of photodamage.

33

The Effect of Topical Tretinoin on Photodamaged Skin Surface Parameters

A. Sparavigna, G. Galbiati, G. Viscardi
Dept. Derm., 'San Gerardo dei Tintori' Hospital, Monza, Italy

In order to evaluate the influence of a 5-month treatment with a 0.025% tretinoin emulsion on surface parameters of photodamaged facial skin, hydration, sebum level, pH and mechanical properties were investigated in treated and nontreated areas of 20 female patients. The measurements were done, under standard conditions, using a 'Skin-tester' (by IMS, Haifa, Israel) for the study of skin capacitance, phototransmittance of sebum and pH and a 'PEC' suction device (by EDS, Bologna, Italy) for the study of mechanical properties, in basal conditions and monthly during the treatment. Comparing the measurements, we obtained the following significant results in the treated areas: increased hydration and elastic recovery, decreased sebum level and pH.

34

Skin Aging Visualization Using Multimedia Image Processing System

F. Mizoguchi[a], *Y. Ohwada*[a], *M. Tanaka*[b], *K. Moroshawa*[b], *M. Takahashi*[b], *Y. Kawajiri*[a]
[a]Science University of Tokyo, Intelligent System Lab., Japan, [b]Shiseido Research Center, Japan

A new information system using multimedia image processing system has been developed for skin aging visualization. This system makes it easier to categorize the real image of skin aging using Fractal geometry which simulates aging patterns of skin. By comparing Fractal patterns with skin aging data from direct skin analyzer, we have extracted the skin aging patterns which were further classified into aging image data. Using Macintosh as multimedia workstation, we implemented for skin aging visualization as the multimedia image processing system. We have adopted two basic methods for this system: one is Fractal geometry using constraint language (Mathematica) and the other is to use image classification the recent artificial intelligence techniques. In this system, we have characterized the skin aging together with the categorized images for each aged generation. The final goal of this system will be indexing using Fractal patterns of skin aging through the real image data analysis.

35

Changes in Skin Line Pattern during Senescence Process Analysed by Fractal Methods and Fourier Transformation

S. Motta[a], *L. Mellesi*[a], *S. Mattiuz*[b], *D. Marini*[b], *M. Monti*[a]
[a]Ist Clinic of Dermatology and [b]Department of Computer Science, University of Milan, Italy

Skin age estimation requires reliable and quasi automatic methods; this paper presents experimental results based on a new methodology of image processing techniques in order to find meaningful parameters capable of characterizing different skin samples. The parameters are computed directly on a digitised image of skin samples without using mechanical instruments. For the discrimination of different classes of skin age, fractal properties of skin texture, correlated with roughness, together with Fourier analysis of digitised image, correlated to anisotropy and density of peaks and furrows were analysed. 90 silicon rubber skin replicas from volar forearm of 90 healthy subjects of both sexes (ranging from 0 to 90 years of age) were collected. The images of skin replica were digitised using a CCD camera, filters were used to eliminate frame distortion and background noise. Then, each replica underwent fractal and power spectrum analysis. According to the parameter results, the specimens were classified by cluster analysis. This automatic classification system produced a partition set of the 90 analysed images in 4 age classes. In order to evaluate the performance of the automatic method we asked five dermatologists to subdivide the 90 replicas in the same 4 classes and compared the objective and the subjective results. This study demonstrates that the ratio between chronologic age and skin texture can be defined and that once defined the range of normality ratio, the study of skin senescence, extrinsic age, diseased and pharmacological premature age will be more precise and accurate.

36

Discrepancies in Mechanical Measurements of Skin in Assessing Ageing

H.G. Vogel
Hoechst, Frankfurt, FRG

Age of an individual is mainly estimated by the appearance of his skin. On the positive side youth is related to a soft skin with high turgor. It seems reasonable to estimate age by measuring mechanical properties of skin. In this respect, many attempts have been made using various methods with contradictory results. Whereas in vitro studies of human and animal skin show quite similar results the comparison between in vitro and in vivo data is possible only on the basis of corrections due to the experimental conditions. Results of in vivo studies on mechanical properties of human skin are rather contradictory. The use of different methods (force perpendicular to the skin surface or horizontal to the skin surface) makes the comparison of the results rather difficult. Reasons for the discrepancies will be discussed. Standardisation of methods is absolutely necessary.

Image Analysis and Other Data Analysis on Ultrasound Recordings

37

From Qualitative to Quantitative Ultrasound: A Difficult Task

B. Querleux
Laboratories de Recherche de L'Oréal, Aulnay-sous-Bois, France

High resolution imaging by ultrasound is becoming a widespread method for in vivo skin investigations. In the past, studies aimed at spatial resolution enhancement in order to be able to measure different skin structures such as skin thickness, epidermis thickness, evaluation of the nonechogenic band of the upper dermis or visualization of pilosebaceous units for instance.

Nowadays there appear more and more studies in which authors report not only important results about a better visualization of skin structures but also report what they call quantitative skin characterization by estimation of acoustical parameters and/or texture analysis through first-order and second-order grey level statistics.

Other research laboratories have already published quantitative ultrasonic characterization on tissues such as liver or muscle in the standard frequency range (1–10 MHz). There is abundant literature about the difficulties of such measurements which necessitate the elimination or at least diminish the influence on the quantified estimations of the features of the system used and more particularly of the transducer. Many methods have been presented which correct the biased estimations, but their validity as well as their usefulness at higher skin frequency range (10–40 MHz) have still to be checked.

This paper tries to illustrate with examples to what extent, for skin quantitation, the influence of the transducer features and the acquisition methods have to be analyzed and in some cases taken into account. Otherwise, quantified results would be unrealistic or at least biased and in any case device-dependent.

38

Age-Dependent Variations of Normal Skin: Image Processing on 20-MHz B Scan Recordings

S. Seidenari, A. Pagnoni, C. Lasagni, A. Giannetti
Department of Dermatology, University of Modena, Italy

Department of Dermatology, University of Modena, Italy 80 subjects of four different age groups were studied by a 20-MHz B scanner of six skin sites. In order to assess echogenicity of the upper and lower part of the skin according to age, image segmentation was performed by dividing the amplitude scale into bands, and by selecting amplitude intervals highlighting the hyper- and hyporeflecting parts of the epidermis and of the dermis and tissue characterized by intermediate echoamplitudes. By this method a great regional variation in the acoustic behaviour of elderly skin with respect to skin of young subjects can be demonstrated. However, a general trend can be identified, consisting in a shift from low intensity of ultrasound echoes, characteristic in the dermis of young subjects, to intermediate or high reflection amplitudes, which are more frequent in elderly skin.

Plenary Session

Assessment of Skin Surface

39

Assessment of Skin Irritation with Bioengineering Techniques

J. Serup
University of Copenhagen, Bispebjerg Hospital (Bioengineering and Skin Research Laboratory) and Leo Pharmaceutical Products (Department of Dermatological Research), Copenhagen, Denmark

Irritant skin reactions are not uniform but dependent on the irritant, its way of penetration into the skin and the specific nature of its toxic effect. In contrast, allergic reactions share the same pathogenetic events, and a comparable phenomenology irrespective of the allergen.

Epidermal changes can be characterized and quantified with skin replica, and from measurements of electrical conductance, electrical capacitance, thermographic imaging of the skin surface, and transepidermal water loss.

The vasodilation can be measured with laser Doppler flowmetry and with different methods for measuring the skin colour. Skin colour measurement reflects the volume of erythrocytes under a given area of skin, and it is strongly depended on the orthostatic position. The flow represents moving erythrocytes and is less dependent on orthostatic position. Measurement of vasodilation is generally sensitive, but the vasodilation is fully developed already in reactions moderate in strengths.

Edema formation can be measured and characterized by the use of a high-frequency ultrasound technique including image analysis of inflammatory band formations in the outer dermis. This band is already visible in weak reactions. Edema formation is as compared to vasodilation more prominent in advanced reactions.

With bioengineering techniques a detailed characterization of skin irritation is possible. Also subclinical changes can be recorded. For example, water itself is under occlusion slightly damaging to the water barrier of the skin.

Bioengineering methods have now reached a position, where they are commonly used in the field of contact dermatitis. It is recommended that a number of methods are used both to cover skin surface changes, vasodilation and edema formation. The level of information is considerably higher with a multiparametric approach.

Mechanical and Electrical Properties of the Skin

40

Mechanical Measurements of Skin

H.G. Vogel
Hoechst, Frankfurt/Main, FRG

The mechanical properties of skin are of interest for various reasons. They are influenced by maturation and ageing as well as by skin diseases. Several methods have been developed to study the biomechanics of skin. In vitro methods, i.e. animal studies with skin samples ex vivo, or studies on human cadaver skin have the advantage to give reliable and reproducible results. Various parameters can be measured by stress-strain experiments, such as skin thickness, tensile strength, ultimate extension and ultimate modulus of elasticity. Under special experimental conditions, such as hysteresis, relaxation, repeated strain and creeping, parameters indicating viscosity and secondary elasticity can be measured. Data obtained from human cadaver skin are in good agreement with results from animal experiments. With some corrections according to the experimental conditions in vitro data can be compared with in vivo results. Animal experiments allowed to study the age dependence of in vivo recovery after repeated strain. Various methods have been used to study the mechanical properties of human skin in vivo by applying forces either perpendicular or horizontal to the skin surface. Unfortunately, the results obtained with different methods are difficult to compare. Therefore standardisation of the methods is highly recommended.

41

Measurement and Analysis of Skin Impedance

Y. Yamamoto
Dept Electrical & Electronic Eng, Okayama University, Japan

Skin impedance is characterized by high impedance due to a high resistance of the stratum corneum and varies dramatically according to measurement and the circumference inside and outside a human body. Therefore, a skin impedance which has many factors is expected on applying various measurement methods. Simultaneously, the same reasons have not made the measurements simple. The circumference factors influencing on skin impedance are as follows: (1) temperature, (2) humidity and (3) style of every day life. The biological and physiological factors affecting skin impedance are as follows: (1) portion, (2) perspiration, (3) body temperature and (4) drugs and cosmetics. The factors relating to measuring conditions are as follows: (1) types of electrode and electrolyte paste (dry or wet, and including electrolyte), (2) time after applying the electrode, (3) frequency and magnitude of electric current or voltage, (4) time during current through and its history. Generally speaking, in case of skin impedance application caution must be taken not or little disturbing the natural conditions. The following has been studied: (1) searching for various diseases inside the body, (2) acupuncture in oriental medicine, (3) detection of dermatological disease, (4) evaluation of the action of drug and cosmetics and (5) diagnosis of psychological disease. The considerations of the problems as the interface in the passing of bioelectrical signals are as follows: (1) hydration and ionic injection decreasing the skin impedance, (2) stripping epidermal stratum corneum, and (3) use of high frequency decreasing the skin impedance.

Blood Circulation

42

Thermography

I. Fujimasa
Research Center for Advanced Science and Technology, The University of Tokyo, Japan

The infrared thermography is a noninvasive measurement method of skin temperature distribution. It has been applied clinically to peripheral vascular diseases, neuromuscular diseases, inflammatory diseases and tumors since 1968. The full-scale application started in the early 1980s with the introduction of computerized image acquisition and processing to thermograph instruments. The image diagnostic principles do not depend upon pattern recognition or statistical analysis seen on other radiographic image diagnoses, but upon quantitative analysis using thermal simulation models of the disease pathophysiologies. The thermatome is a typical image expression to find a thermally abnormal location on skin. To describe a specified pathophysiological phenomenon on a thermographic image, the parameter reduction technics have been developed. Pattern transition caused by individual, sexual, time, seasonal, and other environmental variations are usually eliminated by computer image handling tools. Some kinds of thermatome, such as the blood flow-dependent thermatome, named angiothermatome, autonomic nerve stimulation-dependent thermatome: neurothermatome, muscular blood flow-dependent thermatome: myothermatome, can be described by many kinds of image processing technics, such as asymmetry, time difference, and temperature fluctuation frequency detection. Thermatomes caused by metabolic and inflammatory abnormality are mainly evaluated by thermographic index expression and histogram analysis. Recently, some dynamic analysis methods under stress tests have added to such stationary analysis. Thus, the thermography will become a true dynamic physiological function imaging machine.

43
Cutaneous Blood Flow

P.G. Agache
Department of Dermatology, University of Besançon, France

The skin has a rich vascular supply (1/9 of the heart output while its weight represents only 1/40 to 1/30 of body weight) but with wide regional variations. The vascular pattern is characterized by a segmental supply from muscular arteries and 3 intradermal interconnected plexuses (deep dermis, periadnexal, subepidermal) where the bulk is made of capacitance vessels. Numerous arteriovenous glomi are found in the extremities. In no way is the skin vascular pattern terminal so that skin nonfunction is not possible. At rest skin blood flow largely exceeds the metabolic needs. This is to match prolonged ischemia due to body pressure and thermoregulation. Local and systemic regulation governs the skin blood flow through cytokine secretion, autonomic nervous and hormonal control.

Ultrasound Techniques

44
Ultrasound Examination of Skin Structures

Y. Miki, Y. Watanabe, S. Miyauchi, S. Murakami
Dept. Derm., Univ. Ehime, School Med., Japan

Ultrasound is a noninvasive and real-time diagnostic procedure and can be applied to examine normal and abnormal structures of the skin. In vivo vertical B scan echograms of the skin using 25-, 40- and 60-MHz sector scanners were presented in comparison with the corresponding routine histologic sections. The actual axial and lateral resolutions of the scanners were in the range of about 0.1–0.25 mm, and the depths of the echo penetration were 3.5–1 mm. Discussions on the fundamental problems of the ultrasound application in the skin histology were made on the level of the image resolution and the tissue characterization. A recent application of a three-dimensional reconstruction of the echograms using computer graphics was also presented.

New Bioengineering Techniques II

45
Optical Spectroscopy in Skin

R. Rox Anderson

The advantages and apparent limitations of optical spectroscopy in skin will be discussed. The basis for reflectance, fluorescence, and specialized laser techniques such as coherence, time-resolved, and frequency-domain spectroscopy will be briefly presented. The medical potential for in vivo optical spectroscopy is significant, but not yet well developed. Radiation transport models which specify tissue reflectance and fluorescence in terms of the intrinsic parameters μa (absorption coefficient), $\mu s'$ (reduced scattering coefficient) and μf (fluorescence coefficient) will be reviewed. The role of optical spectroscopy in administration of photodynamic therapy (PDT) for cancer is critical, and will be used as an example. Detection of PDT drug (benzoporphyrin derivative) concentration in tissue can be made either by reflectance or fluorescence, and yields pharmacokinetic information. Irreversible photobleaching of PDT drugs, and partial consumption of oxygen though photochemical reactions, can both be monitored noninvasively. In addition, response of tissue to PDT, including Hb oxygen saturation and blood content have been measured with a versatile diode-array spectroreflectometer. Recent measurements of autofluorescence spectra from living human and mouse skin will also be presented. Resolution of these spectra into six discrete excitation-emission bands will be presented, related to various epidermal and dermal fluorophores.

46
Cutaneous pO_2 and pCO_2

H. Takiwaki
Department of Dermatology, School of Medicine, University of Tokushima, Japan

Transcutaneous partial pressure of oxygen ($tcpO_2$) and carbon dioxide ($tcpCO_2$) represent partial pressures of these two gasses measured on the surface of the skin. Since the tested site is occluded and heated by the probe head with a built-in heater in the usual way, not only the flux of CO_2 but also that of O_2 arise from the inside of the skin to the outside. Once the steady state has been achieved, the $tcpO_2$ and $tcpCO_2$ show good correlations with the arterial pO_2 and pCO_2, respectively, and quickly respond to their changes. The method, therefore, is widely being utilized to monitor the arterial pO_2 and pCO_2 noninvasively. However, $tcpO_2$ and $tcpCO_2$ are also influenced by various cutaneous factors like cellular respiration and permeability of gasses in the skin. Thus, if arterial pO_2 and pCO_2 are normal while $tcpO_2$ and/or $tcpCO_2$ are not, the cause is likely to lie in the skin tested. To our knowledge, $tcpO_2$ decreases more or less in many skin lesions with pathological changes such as hyperkeratosis, acanthosis, cellular infiltration, fibrosis and so on. $tcpCO_2$ is rather stable in such conditions, but extremely high values are recorded when prenecrotic changes appear in the skin.

Photoaging and Race

47
Noninvasive Methods for Assessing the Physiologic and Structural Changes in Photodamaged Human Skin

Albert M. Kligman
Department of Dermatology, University of Pennsylvania, School of Medicine, Philadelphia, Pa., USA

Actinically damaged skin is easily recognized in older individuals who show wrinkles, mottling, laxity, dryness, follicular impactions, and uneven texture.

There is a need to obtain more objective assessments of the degree of photodegradation. This would be especially valuable for determining the therapeutic benefits of surgical interventions such as chemical peels and corrective drugs such as retinoids.

The abnormalities of photoaged facial skin are numerous and diverse. Hence, a battery of tests are required to establish a quantitative profile.

The procedures to be demonstrated include: (1) ultraviolet photography, (2) photography by polarized light, (3) cyanoacrylate follicular biopsies, (4) adhesive discs (D'Squames) to determine degree of occult scaling, (5) exfoliative cytology (sticky slides and detergent scrubs), (6) nicotinate stimulated blood flow (laser Doppler), (7) dansyl chloride stratum corneum turnover, (8) microtopography of corneocytes by scanning electron microscopy and (9) surface glyphic patterns using shadowed Silflo replicas.

48
Racial Differences in Skin Function

E. Berardesca
Department of Dermatology, University of Pavia, IRCCS Policlinico S. Matteo, Pavia, Italy

Skin color and melanin content are the most important differences characterizing racial groups. Several parameters related to skin function have been investigated noninvasively to correlate skin physiology and pigmentation. Marked differences exist among races and are related to the protective role of melanin present in darker skin. Pigmentation affects mainly skin mechanical properties. Skin color also seems to modulate irritant and vascular reactions: blacks and whites show a different proclivity to developing erythema and barrier function damage after exposure to surfactants.

49

Non-Invasive Assessment of Biaxial Young's Modulus of Man in vivo

P.G. Agache[a], *D. Varchon*[b], *Ph. Humbert*[a], *A. Rochefort*[a]
[a]Department of Dermatology and [b]Department of Applied Mechanics, University of Besançon, France

The elastic modulus (E) is a major parameter of the skin mechanical behaviour. Unfortunately up to now only its variation could be currently estimated in vivo, and without access to absolute differences. Using a suction device and ultrasonic measurement of skin thickness (skin imaging at 25 MHz), and a modelling of deformation, we could assess the E value of the volar forearm skin (epidermis + dermis) in vivo. With a 20-mm diameter cup and 200-mbar depression, the E value in 53 healthy subjects was 76 ± 62 kPa and very asymmetrical in distribution. The height of skin lifting was 0.49 ± 0.16 mm and skin thickness 1.039 ± 0.122 mm. Previously on a small number of subjects E had been found independent of the cup diameter (2 or 4 or 6 mm) and of the depression (100 or 200 mbar). The model offers the possibility of current assessment of the absolute value of E in vivo in a simple and non-invasive way and might be useful for further insight into the mechanical behaviour of human skin.

50

Skin Elasticity of Systemic Scleroderma

K. Dempo, T. Sasaki, H. Nakajima
Department of Dermatology, Yokohama City University School of Medicine, Japan

Objective. Skin elasticity was measured with an advanced noninvasive skin elasticity measurement in 29 patients with systemic scleroderma (PSS) and 13 controls.

Methods. Repeated suction was applied to a 75-mm^2 circular skin area, and tensile distensibility, hysteresis (H) and resilient distension (RD) were measured.

Results. H and RD of the PSS skin were decreased compared with those of the controls.

Conclusion. These results suggest that skin elasticity measurement with this instrument will be useful in objectively assessing the stiffness of skin afflicted with PSS.

51

A Pocket Size Skin Admittance Meter with Three-Electrode System and Lock-In Technique

Ø. Martinsen[a, b], *S. Grimnes*[b], *J. Karlsen*[a]
[a]Biotechnology Centre of Oslo, and [b]Department of Physics, University of Oslo, Norway

Commercial lock-in amplifiers used for skin conductance and susceptance measurements are bulky devices, and only suitable for laboratory use. Furthermore, they must be modified to enable use of the three-electrode system.

A pocket size instrument is presented for measurements outside the laboratory and for protracted admittance recordings in the subjects' normal environment, when connected to a small data logger. Our intention is primarily to use the instrument to investigate the effect of topical preparations on human skin.

The instrument is implemented with a quadrature-oscillator, supplying the three-electrode system with a sine-voltage and the two lock-in amplifiers with a sine and cosine reference signal. The oscillator frequency is determined by the values of four resistors in a plug-in unit, and is easily changed by replacement of this unit. The current through the measuring electrode is converted to a voltage with a transresistance amplifier, and errors caused by the use of shunt resistor are therefore avoided. Any 50/60 Hz noise, caused by stray capacitance between the test subject and power lines, is also eliminated by the three-electrode system. Comparators convert the reference signals into square waves that are used to gate the switches in the lock-in amplifiers. The flanks of the square waves can be calibrated individually. When the voltage of one of the two 9-volt power supply batteries drops below a preset value, the measurements are interrupted and an LED is lit on the front panel. Adjustable offset and gain on the output amplifiers make it possible to connect the instrument to a variety of devices, such as voltmeters, data loggers, X-Y plotters, A/D converters, etc.

52

Measurements of Skin Elasticity with a New Suction Device – Relation to Age, Sex, and Anatomical Region in Normal Skin and Its Comparison with Some Diseased Skin

M. Nishimura, T. Tsuji
Department of Dermatology, Nagoya City University Medical School, Japan

Using a recently developed in vivo suction device for measuring skin elasticity, we evaluated age, sex and regional (sun-exposed or nonexposed) differences in the elastic properties. Skin elasticity was decreased with aging at all anatomical regions examined. Differences between the regions were significant in the same age groups, but not between the sexes. In some skin diseases (PSS and Ehlers-Danlos syndrome) skin elasticity showed a characteristic abnormality when compared with age- and region-matched normal skin. This procedure allows assessment of skin elasticity, and its application to diseased skin, particularly connective tissue disorders may be helpful for diagnosing, deciding progression and evaluating therapeutic effects.

53

Development of a Stiffness Meter for the Skin Surface

H. Oka[a], *T. Yamamoto*[a], *T. Kajikawa*[b], *N. Narahashi*[b]
[a]Fac. Eng. Okayama Univ., Japan;
[b]Shiseido Inst. Beauty Sciences, Tokyo, Japan

Biomechanical properties of skin surface are measured in clinics, skin science, cosmetics, etc. A quantification can also be made by palpation, pressation and percussion. The authors have developed a measurement system which can obtain a biomechanical impedance by applying a random vibration onto the human body. The system, however, is fairly large in scale, because it contains a personal computer which is used for data calculation and analysis. A new stiffness meter is introduced applying a single sinusoidal vibration onto the skin surface. By adopting a single sinusoidal vibration both the software and the hardware of the measuring system are simplified. The stiffness meter is characterized by a portable size and rapid measurement, and it resembles a clinical instrument.

A sinusoidal vibration (≑ 250 Hz) is applied to the human body and an acceleration at the same driving point is detected by using the measuring probe. The measuring probe uses the bimorph piezoelectric ceramics. We adopt one ceramic of the probe for driving and another for detecting an acceleration. When the preload onto the skin surface becomes the initial set preload, the measurement of the acceleration is automatically executed. We propose a new index, SH, which is a value of panel counter corresponding to 1/A. Though the SH value is an index of skin stiffness, it has physical meanings in proportion to biomechanical impedance. Because a reciprocal of acceleration (A) is in proportion to a mechanical impedance, when driving force and frequency are constant, it is possible to evaluate the stiffness of body surface by using SH. The measurement repeatability of the stiffness meter is 2%.

54

Comparison of Irritancy of Shampoo Using Normal Human Keratinocyte Culture Model and Laser Doppler Blood Flow Measurement

Hee Chul Eun, Hyung Chan Pyo, Seoung Young Chung
Department of Dermatology, College of Medicine, Seoul National University, Korea

Shampoos are commonly used cosmetics in daily life and can cause irritant dermatitis in high concentrations. For the evaluation of skin irritancy, keratinocyte culture is used as well as noninvasive techniques including laser Doppler blood flow measurement. Shampoo is one of the ideal finished products for which the cell culture cytotoxicity technique can be useful. We have compared in vivo laser Doppler blood flow measurement of patch test responses to several shampoos with in vitro keratinocyte cell culture irritancy measured by MTT and lactic dehydrogenase activity after adding the same shampoos in various concentrations.

Our data showed that there is a relatively good correlation between these two models.

55

Effects of a Soya-Based Bath Oil on Transepidermal Water Loss in Severe Atopic Dermatitis

G. Borroni, C. Zaccone, G. Vignati, G.P. Vignoli, E. Berardesca, G. Rabbiosi
Department of Human and Hereditary Pathology, Institute of Dermatology, University of Pavia and IRCCS Policlinico S. Matteo, Pavia, Italy

Atopic skin is frequently characterized by dryness, even in uninvolved skin. In the last decade, several experimental studies in atopic skin demonstrated impairment in barrier function and skin hygroscopicity. Correct detersion is of no little significance with atopic dermatitis; in fact, aggressive surfactants or excessive washing may induce further dehydration. The effects of a bath oil containing soya oil (82.95%) on transepidermal water loss (TEWL) were studied both in a group of patients with severe atopic dermatitis (AD) and in a control group. Measurements were carried out on the volar forearms, using the Evaporimeter EP 1 (ServoMed, Stockholm, Sweden). After basal measurements, the right forearm was immersed in a solution of the bath oil in water at 37 °C for 5 min; the left forearm was immersed in water and acted as a control. Evaporimeter measurements were taken at 1, 5, 15, 30 and 60 min after the skin was dried. The control group failed to show any differences between the sites tested at any of the measurement times. On the other hand, AD patients showed a significant reduction ($p < 0.05$) in TEWL on the treated forearm at 60 min (6.93 vs. 9.05). Our results show that the bath oil tested is a useful aid in modulating TEWL in AD patients.

56

The Sorption-Desorption Test in the Evaluation of Skin Hygroscopicity in Physiological and Pathological Conditions

G. Borroni, G. Vignati, C. Zaccone, G.P. Vignoli, E. Berardesca, G. Rabbiosi
Department of Human and Hereditary Pathology, Institute of Dermatology, University of Pavia and IRCCS Policlinico S. Matteo, Pavia, Italy

The sorption-desorption test is a useful tool in the evaluation of the kinetics of skin hydration in physiological and pathological conditions. This test is based on the recording of the electrical properties of stratum corneum (impedance, capacitance) before and after the application of water on the skin. Extracellular lipids of the stratum corneum play an important role in regulating its water content. The aim of this work was to evaluate the hygroscopicity of stratum corneum after delipidization and following skin irritation induced by surfactants. A Corneometer CM 820 PC (Courage Khazaka, Köln, FRG) was used. Fourteen healthy subjects (mean age 31.3 ± 4.5) were studied on 4 different sites on the volar forearms. A basal measurement was taken; site 1 and site 2 were then delipidized, the former using acetone/ether (1:1) for 5 min and the latter using chloroform/ethanol (2:1) for 3 min; site 3 was exposed to sodium lauryl sulphate 5% for 5 min; site 4 was bathed with water for 5 min and acted as a control site. After contact with these substances was stopped, each site was bathed in water for 30 s, corneometer measurements were then recorded every 30 s for 10 min, then every 2 min for a further 10 min, finally every 5 min for a further 10 min. The data recorded in this study showed that delipidization obtained using solvents induces a decrease in the hygroscopicity of stratum corneum; significant dehydration was seen following both acetone/ether and chloroform/ethanol; it appeared early and was still present at 30 min. The implications of these findings are discussed.

57

Water Removal from the Body during Hemodialysis: Effects on Some Skin Biophysical Parameters

V. Brazzelli[a], G.P. Vignoli[a], G. Borroni[a], A. Cavagnino[b], E. Berardesca[a]
[a]Department of Dermatology, University of Pavia, Policlinico S. Matteo, Italy;
[b]Hemodialysis Center, Borgomanero, Italy

Water plays an important role in maintaining skin suppleness and elasticity. We used hemodialysis as a model to investigate the effects on biophysical properties of the skin induced by removal of fluids and water from the body. The following parameters have been investigated before and immediately after a hemodialytic session: body weight, skin elasticity and distensibility, skin hydration, TEWL and skin thickness. A significant decrease was recorded after treatment in body weight, skin thickness ($p < 0.01$) and skin elasticity ($p < 0.01$). Significant linear correlations were found between stratum corneum water content, skin distensibility and TEWL.

The data reveal that rapid removal of body fluids influences skin biophysical properties: early changes in skin thickness and ground substance occur in the dermis and affect mechanical properties of the skin. The decrease of water content in the upper layers of the skin occurs at a later stage and influences skin hydration rather than TEWL. This model is a useful tool to investigate water kinetics through the skin.

58

Skin Surface Lipids and Water Content of the Horny Layer of Children's Face

C. Kuwahara[a], *Y. Aaraya*[a], *Y. Ogino*[b], *K. Arisu*[b], *R. Hayakawa*[b]
[a] Research and Development Department, PIGEON Corporation Laboratory, Tsukuba, Japan; [b] Division of Dermatology, Nagoya University Branch Hospital, Japan

In order to obtain elementary data for a correct skin care of the child, we examined the amount of skin surface lipids and water content of the horny layer of children's face. The data of the children were compared to those of healthy adults. The subjects were 51 newborn babies, 24 1-month-old babies, 23 infants aged from 3 months to 2 years and 8 months and 30 healthy adults (17 males and 13 females).

The amount of water content of the horny layer was measured with a skin surface hygrometer (SKICON-200; IBS). The amount of skin surface lipids was measured with a lipid meter (RICOH). The amount of skin surface lipids of children was significantly ($p < 0.01$) lower than that of the healthy adults. In particular, the skin surface lipids of the infant group aged from 3 months to 2 years and 8 months were remarkably lower than those of the others. The water content of the horny layer of children was nearly the same as that of the healthy adults.

From the above results, we thought the main cause of dry skin of children was due to the deficiency of the skin surface lipids. We concluded that the children's face should not be washed with strong soaps or detergents and they should be treated with moisturizing creams rich in oil.

59

Quantitation of Sweat Using the Skin Surface Hygrometer and Its Application

S.H. Lee[a], *W. Hur*[b], *S.K. Ahn*[b], *W.H. Kang*[b]
[a] Department of Dermatology, Yonsei University College of Medicine, Seoul, Korea; [b] Department of Dermatology, Yonsei University Wonju College of Medicine, Wonju, Korea

Sweat on the surface of skin may alter the hydration state of the stratum corneum. The altered amount of hydration on skin surface after sweating may reflect the quantity of the delivered sweat indirectly. The skin surface hygrometer which was introduced by Tagami (1982) can measure the hydration state of the skin surface quickly and quantitatively.

In this study, as a first step, we investigated the role of sweating on the hydration state in stratum corneum by measurement of altered conductance of the electric current using the skin surface hygrometer (SKICON 200, IBS, Japan) after stimulation or blocking the sweat glands. As a next step, in order to investigate the pharmacologic responsiveness of sweat glands in psoriasis and localized scleroderma, we applied this method for quantitation of sweating using the skin surface hygrometer.

In this study we have demonstrated that (1) sweating is one of the factors to determine the hydration state of stratum corneum and (2) the functional abnormalities in the development of sweat secretion in the lesions of psoriasis and morphea could be involved in the pathogenesis of these diseases.

60

Application of a Special Electrical Property Measurement Protocol to Lips

D.L. Miller
bioNET, Dallas, Tex., USA

A protocol was devised that generated both moisture level and rate of moisture loss data from a single 10-second measurement sequence using a commercially available skin electrical property measuring device. Measurements were made with the NOVA DPM 9003 instrument which produces an output proportional to the skin electrical capacitance in the MHz frequency range. The specially designed probe consisted of concentric circular electrodes with 6 mm outside diameter. Data acquisition was software-controlled using a SHARP laptop PC. Linear regression of the readings taken during the 10-second contact time reduced the data to a slope, SE (rate of signal change with time) and intercept, IE (signal at t = 0). Thus IE was interpreted as indicating the typical moisture content of the surface, *unaffected by the probe.* SE was interpreted as indicating the rate of moisture build-up due to the occlusive presence of the probe, a process initially dependent on the *rate of moisture loss from the surface.* Measurements of treated and untreated lip surfaces were made over several hours after application of a commercial lipstick. Data was taken before and after blotting the product off the lips. Before blotting IE was increased by treatment (more moisture) and SE was decreased (lipstick moisture barrier effect). After blotting, IE remained increased by treatment but SE returned to untreated levels (removal of lipstick barrier effect).

61

The Effect of Kampoh (Japanese-Chinese Traditional Herbal Medicine) Bath Therapy on the Hydration and the Water-Holding Capacity in Atopic Skin

T. Seki, M. Toyoda, M. Morohashi
Department of Dermatology, Faculty of Medicine, Toyama Medical and Pharmaceutical University, Japan

We have already reported that Jio *(Rehmanniae radix)* and Toki *(Angelicae radix)* have the possibility of increasing the epidermal lipogenesis. Epidermal or intercellular lipids of stratum corneum are thought to be one of the main factors to maintain the water holding capacity of the stratum corneum. Hydration and water-holding capacity of stratum corneum are reorted to be lower in atopic patients than that of normal healthy persons. We used the decoctions of Jio and Toki in the bath therapy for patients with atopic dermatitis.

Jio (2 g) and Toki (2 g) were put in 600 ml of water which was brought to boil and then simmered for 30 min. The decocted extracts were then put into a bathtub with 200 liters of comfortably hot water. Fifty-five patients with atopic dermatitis (mean age 8.1 years, range 1–33 years; 30 male, 25 female) had this bath therapy once a day for 6 weeks. Hydration and water-holding capacity of stratum corneum were measured with a skin surface hygrometer (Skikon 200, IBS) every 2 weeks for 6 weeks.

Hydration and water-holding capacity of the stratum corneum at 6 weeks after treatment were statistically ($p < 0.01$) increased as compared with the data before treatment. A favorable clinical response was achieved in 74.5% of patients with this therapy.

We consider that this Kampoh bath therapy will be helpful as a new additional therapy for atopic dermatitis.

62

In vivo Evaluation of Skin Ageing: Relations between Viscoelastic Properties and Skin Surface Roughness Parameters

A. Barel, P. Clarys
Algemene en Biologische Scheikunde, Vrije Universiteit Brussel, Brussels, Belgium

Ageing of the skin is clearly characterized by changes in a variety of physical parameters related to the dermis. We have studied the influence of age on the mechanical properties of the skin and on skin roughness. Both physical properties are correlated with modifications in the structure of the papillary and reticular dermis.

Viscoelastic properties were determined from the deformation of the skin after a suction is applied on the skin surface (suction method, Cutometer®). From the deformation-time curves and from the stress-strain curves various parameters such as extensibility, recovery, elasticity and Young's modulus were computed.

Skin anisotropy data and skin surface roughness parameters were obtained by visual score of the silicone replicas and from stylus surfometry on the positive epoxy replicas. Measurements were carried out at unexposed skin areas (forearm and thigh) and at sun-exposed areas (face, crow's feet) on a population divided into different age groups.

In agreement with previous published data significant differences were observed for viscoelastic and skin roughness parameters between some age groups. Both physical parameters are strongly related and appear to be a reliable and objective assessment of skin ageing.

63

High Echography Resolution of the Skin: Principles and Results

S. Diridollou[a], *Y. Gall*[a], *M. Berson*[b], *A. Roncin*[b], *L. Pourcelot*[b]
[a] Centre Jean-Louis Alibert, Pierre Fabre Cosmétique, Vigoulet-Auzil, France; [b] Laboratoire de Biophysique Médicale, Faculté de Medecine, Tours, France

The method is based on a remote measurement betwen an ultrasound transducer (working at 20 MHz) and the more or less deformed cutaneous surface by a technique of suction.

This device enables us to study the static and dynamic behaviour of the cutaneous coating and to quantify its rheologic properties in physiological and pathological conditions. It measures certain dermal alterations as well as the efficiency of their therapeutics.

In dermatology, it can be a good means for studying the effects and the efficiency of cosmetics on the skin towards external aggressions and cutaneous ageing.

64

Echographic Evaluation of Irritant Reactions Induced by Nonanoic Acid, Hydrochloric Acid and Sodium Lauryl Sulfate: A Comparison with TEWL Assessment

S. Seidenari, A. Di Nardo, E. Schiavi, P. Pepe
Department of Dermatology, University of Modena, Italy

On 18 healthy patients patch tests with nonanoic acid 40%, hydrochloric acid 4%, and sodium lauryl sulfate 3% were performed on the volar aspect of the forearm with a 24-hour application time. Evaluation of skin reactions was performed by evaporimetry and by echography. 20-MHz B scan recordings were processed by a dedicated program, which ascribed an arbitrary scale to the amplitude values of the echoes and was able to give a numerical representation to image data. Pictures were evaluated by an ultrasound amplitude band, ranging from 0 to 30, marking hyporeflecting parts of the tissue (corresponding to edema and inflammatory infiltration) and by a 201–255 band, highlighting hyperreflecting parts of the image (epidermis). By using this method a characteristic echographic pattern can be demonstrated for different irritants. Values of hyper- and hyporeflecting pixels can be correlated to TEWL measurements.

65

Ultrasonic Analysis of Microparticles Injected into Guinea Pig Skin

M. Shimozuma[a], *H. Nakagawa*[b], *Y. Ishibashi*[b]
[a] Department of Dermatology, Kosei General Hospital, and [b] Department of Dermatology, University of Tokyo, Tokyo, Japan

It is an advantage for dermatologists to be able to employ ultrasonic equipment with high frequency and high resolution to investigate skin lesions located in the superficial parts of the body. But, with higher resolution, we often encounter difficulties in comparing ultrasonic images with histopathological findings because of the possible changes of microstructure of the tissue after excision and fixation.

We used polysthylene particles to evaluate the ultrasonic images of microstructure in vivo, because they are supposed to remain unchanged in the tissue. Polysthylene particles ranging from 1 to 30 μm were injected into the dorsal skin of guinea pigs. A 30-MHz ultrasonic equipment with axial 120 μm and lateral 160 μm resolution was used to analyze ultrasonic images of the particles. The particles with a diameter of 20–30 μm were detectable as hyperechoic mass, while the particles with a diameter of 1 and 10 μm were not detectable as clear images. The size of the components between 10 and 20 μm was a critical factor.

This experimental model may be useful to understand ultrasonic images of skin lesions on the basis of microstructure.

66

Surface Microscopy of Pigmented Skin Lesions

R. Akasu, H. Sugiyama, A. Osada, C. Akiyama, A. Saitoh, K. Tsukamoto, N. Ohtake, O. Takayama, M. Furue, K. Tamaki
Yamanashi Medical College, Dept. Derm., Yamanashi, Japan

Observation of pigmented lesions with a stereomicroscope after application of immersion oil to the skin surface is described. We studied the surface microscopic features of nevocellular nevi (NCN), basal cell carcinomas (BCC), blue nevi, seborrheic keratoses, solar lentigines and malignant melanomas (MM) with a dermatoscope (Heine Delta-10, FRG). The surface microscopic data were correlated with histological features on serial step sections.

NCN showed homogeneous brown to black pigmentation and gray globules were seen in some cases. Blue nevi were relatively well-demarcated homogeneous steel blue pigmentation. BCCs were seen with the dermatoscope to be characterized by waxy nodules covered by atrophic epidermis. Telangiectasia was also found in most cases. Circular white areas (pseudohorn cysts) were the characteristic features of seborrheic keratoses and honey comb-like pigment networks of solar lentigines. MM showed a pigment pattern which varied from dark brown to steel blue. White depigmentation and bizarre looking black dots were also features. Moreover, we also studied pigment moles on soles using a monitor microscope (VH-5910, Keyence, Japan) which can magnify the surface up to 500×. Patterns of pigmentation were classified into several types and histological features corresponding to these types were also discussed.

67

New Objective Methods for Assessment of Skin Pigmentation

N. Ando[a, b], *C. Edwards*[b], *R. Marks*[b]
[a]POLA Labs, Japan, [b]Department of Dermatology, University of Wales College of Medicine, Cardiff, UK

Skin colour is major descriptive parameter in clinical and photobiological research, but it is difficult to obtain a precise description of skin colour when evaluating changes in pigmentation.

We have developed two new objective methods for quantifying pigmentation. These involve measuring the diffuse reflectance of skin and the melanin content of surface corneocytes.

An exposed and a non-exposed site were studied in 24 volunteers. First a reflectance spectrometric instrument, the melanin index meter, was used to measure an optical melanin index (OMI) from each site. Then from the same sites a layer of corneocytes was obtained by the adhesive tape stripping method. The percentage of corneocyte area occupied by melanin granules was measured using image analysis as the surface melanin index (SMI). Finally a 4-mm punch biopsy was taken and stained to show dopa-positive cells, indicating active melanin synthesis. The ratio of these cells to the non-stained basal cells gave the histological melanin index (HMI).

Comparison	Non-exposed site	Exposed site
OMI vs. SMI	r = 0.81	r = 0.76
OMI vs. HMI	r = 0.80	r = 0.44
SMI vs. HMI	r = 0.74	r = 0.36

Measurements from the non-exposed site show linear relationships between the three methods, so that either non-invasive method could be used to infer the number of the basal layer melanocytes. However, on the exposed site there is a lower correlation between these methods and the histological method. This could be due to the localisation to the basal layer of dopa-positive melanocytes induced by UV exposure. We conclude that our non-invasive measurements are both reliable in the assessment of skin pigmentation and of local melanin synthesis, and could prove very useful not only in the study of skin colour but also in the assessment of epidermal dyschromia.

68

Measurement of UV Erythema Induced by UVB and PUVA

A. Ogawa, M. Maruyama, H. Tokushige, F. Ogata, Y. Todoroki, S. Moriya, K. Toda
Dept. Derm., Hosp. Tokyo Teishin, Japan

Erythema is the most conspicuous acute cutaneous response to UV radiation. It is a result of an increase in the volume of blood present in the superficial and deep vascular plexi in the dermis, which is visible to the eye. The minimum erythema dose (MED) is defined as the minimum UV radiation dose that produces clearly marginated erythema in the irradiated site, given as a single exposure. In the same way, the minimal phototoxic dose (MPD) is defined as the minimal dose of UVA after ingestion of 8-MOP.

The purpose of this investigation was to find out the most useful and the clinically easiest method to measure the reaction of erythema. Of the erythema 3 × MED induced by UVB and 3 × MPD induced by PUVA, the skin surface temperature was measured by thermography, the deep skin temperature with a deep body thermometer and the skin blood flow with a laser Doppler flowmeter. Our results suggested, of the three methods, the deep skin temperature appeared to correlate best with the clinical observation of erythema reaction induced by UVB and topical PUVA.

69

Analysis of Skin Color Using a Videomicroscope with Computer: The First Step to Differentiate Skin Lesions Automatically

H. Takiwaki, Y. Watanabe, M. Utsunomiya, S. Shirai, K. Nakagawa, Y. Kanno
Department of Dermatology, School of Medicine, University of Tokushima, Japan

We introduce a method for quantified analysis of skin color with a flexible videomicroscope (Dermascope®) connected to a computer. By using indexes derived from absorbance-like values, which were calculated with the mean brightness of the picture picked up in each red, green and blue band, skin color under various conditions was investigated.

At first, we defined indexes for the gradation of erythema and pigmentation. They were linearly correlated with the concentration of oxyhemoglobin and melanin solution in in vitro examination. They also showed correlations with the erythema index and the melanin index by the narrow-band reflectance spectrometer (Dermaspectrometer®) in strongly linear fashions when UV-induced erythema and pigmentation were measured. This system, therefore, can be applied to the semiquantitative evaluation of skin color although the CCD camera mounted is not designed for the exact color measurement.

We further developed a simple computer program to differentiate between lesional skin color automatically, based upon the difference of indexes between a lesion and the adjacent normal skin. About twenty types of lesional skin color were classified by this program, and the correct or meaningful 'instrumental diagnosis' was obtained in about 80% of lesions tested, though they were limited so far to those which showed uniform color.

70

Comparison of Skin pH in Tinea Patients and Control Subjects

K. Chikakane[a], *H. Noguchi*[a], *M. Hiruma*[a], *A. Ishibashi*[a], *H. Takahashi*[b]
[a] Department of Dermatology, National Defense Medical College, Saitama, Japan [b] Department of Dermatology, Teikyo University, School of Medicine, Tokyo, Japan

The skin surface pH on the interdigital spaces of the feet and hands of 69 tinea patients and 19 control subjects was measured. The average skin surface pH of tinea pedis patients' feet and hands was 6.1 and 5.2, respectively. The pH of control subjects' feet and hands was 5.2 and 4.9, respectively. The pH of tinea patients' feet was significantly higher than that of control subjects' feet and tinea patients' hands. The difference was statistically significant. No differences were found between sex and coexistent tinea unguium. Tinea pedis is more frequently seen than tinea manuum. There might be some relationship between tinea frequency and skin pH on the feet and hands. We also compared ammonia on the interdigital spaces of the feet and hands of the other subjects. The skin surface ammonia of the feet was higher than that of the hands.

71

Instrumental Evaluations of Noncationic Materials Derived from Amino Acids as Hair Conditioning Agents

T. Kitano, Y. Kawasaki, K. Sakamoto
Central Research Laboratories, Ajinomoto, Kawasaki, Japan

We have developed reliable and convenient methods to evaluate the efficacy of hair care products. One involves measuring electrostaticity generated through combing with a comb electrode, and the other measuring the frictional coefficient of hair surface with a friction tester. Reproducibility and sensitivity of these methods to substantiate hair care products had been reported previously and efficacy of cationic surfactant as hair conditioning agent has been proven.

In this report, we will discuss the efficacy of three different types of noncationic amino acid derivatives as conditioning agents for hair in comparison with quaternary ammonium chloride. Test articles are as follows: sodium pyrrolidone carboxylate (Na-PCA), Nlauroyl-*L*-lysine (Amihope LL) and PCA ester of glyceryl monooleate (Amifat P-30). These three materials show excellent conditioning effects which are compatible to a cationic surfactant such as quaternary ammonium chloride.

Although it is not a piece of evidence for these effects, it can be speculated that the affinity of these materials to the keratin plays an important role, because these structures have amide bonds which are the same as the protein structure.

Application of amino acid derivatives to hair care formulations would be beneficial not only because of the efficiency mentioned above, but also because of high safety to the skin and the eye mucosa.

72

Measuring the Area of Vitiligo Skin by Computer

E. Masai[a], *M. Ichihashi*[b], *S. Takahashi*[c]
[a]Department of Hygiene, School of Medicine, Kobe University, [b]Department of Dermatology, School of Medicine, Kobe University and [c]Mitsubishi Heavy Industries, Kobe Shipyard and Machinery Works, Kobe, Japan

We have constructed a color PACS (picture archiving and communications system) for dermatology clinics. The system consists of a TV camera, a digitizer of the TV signals, computers, a magnet-optical disk and LAN (local area network). The photographs of the diseased skin are taken by a TV camera and stored in the magnetooptical disk by digitizing the analogue signals of the image from the TV camera. The image data are recorded in the database with the related clinical records that include the important parts of the conventional clinical findings on the paper such as the patient's name and address, diagnosis and the date when the image was taken.

The clinical record in the database constructed in the server computer is easily retrieved by the patient's name, ID number and diagnosis. After that, we can retrieve the image data of the patient by clicking or pushing the button area of the clinical record displayed on the monitor. The server and the clients are connected by the EatherNet. Each client can make its access to the server and retrieve clinical records and image data.

At the moment, the color analyzing program is being developed and installed into the color PACS system. With this program the outline of vitiligo can be defined and the area surrounded by the outline measured.

73

Study of Antimicrobial Efficacy of Hand Washing with an Implement Capable of Quick-Drying: Using Computerized Image Analysis

K. Mitsuya[a], *S. Namura*[a], *S. Nishijima*[a], *Y. Asada*[a], *T. Hatta*[b], *T. Yonekura*[b]
[a]Dept. Derm., Kansai Med. Univ., Moriguchi, Japan; [b]Mitani Co. Toyoshima, Fukui, Japan

We studied the antimicrobial efficacy of hand washing by a quick dry hand washing machine with an ultrasonic wave spraying method. 10 men participated in this study; they pressed their hands on the agar before and after washing hands. And after 48 h incubation at 37 °C, the [ASPECT] of image processing system. When the colonies before hand washing are expressed as 100, those after hand washing are presented as percent reduction. Two patterns of hand washing were carried out in this study: (1) 3 s hand washing using an alcoholic product, Aroclin® and (2) 30 s hand washing using a nonmedicated detergent soap with running water and then washing hands as described in (1).

Advantage of this method: (1) Easy to use for a judgement of antimicrobial efficacy of hand washing, (2) possible to deal with a lot of subjects in a short time and (3) not necessary to use a complicated method.

Disadvantage of this method: (1) Necessary to use a computer (somewhat expensive) and (2) costly to produce medium.

74

Skin Surface Lipids and Water Content of the Horny Layer – In Relation to Sex, Age and Skin Disease

Y. Ogino[a], *R. Hayakawa*[a], *M. Suzuki*[a], *K. Matsunaga*[b], *Y. Arima*[c], *R. Hata*[c], *Y. Otsu*[c]
[a]Div. Derm. Nagoya Univ. Branch Hosp., Nagoya, Japan: [b]Dept. Derm. Fujita Health Univ., Toyoake, Japan; [c]Otsuka Otsu Research Lab., Otsu, Japan

To study the relevance of sex, age and skin diseases to the skin surface lipid and water content of the horny layer, we examined 251 outpatients of our clinic from January to March 1989. The 251 subjects were composed of 21 males and 230 females aged over 16 years. The age distribution of the subjects was 48 teens, 108 in their twenties, 35 thirties, 29 forties, 21 fifties, 7 sixties and 3 seventies. The skin disorders were 105 acne vulgaris, 32 atopic dermatitis, 64 contact dermatitis and 50 other skin diseases. The skin surface lipids were measured with a lipid meter (Ricoh, Shiseido). The water content of the horny layer was measured with a skin surface hygrometer (SKICON-200: IBS). The skin surface lipids of females aged over forty years remarkably decreased compared with those of females under forty. In contrast, in males, we observed no change of skin surface lipid levels in relation to the age brackets. Changes of the water content of the horny layer were neither found in males nor in females.

To discuss the data in relation to skin diseases, we analyzed 134 female patients under forty years since the subject numbers were large enough in each age group. The skin surface lipid level of acne patients was significantly ($p < 0.05$) higher than that of the other diseases. The water content of the horny layer of atopic dermatitis was significantly ($p < 0.05$) lower than that of the other diseases.

Announcement

Prediction of Percutaneous Penetration

Methods Measurements Modelling
Third International Conference

14–16 April 1993
La Grande Motte (Montpellier), France

The Third Prediction of Percutaneous Penetration Conference will take place at the Palais des Congrès, La Grande Motte (Montpellier), France, from 14th to 16th April, 1993. It will provide a dedicated forum for discussion of the latest information on the penetration of compounds through skin and will therefore be of particular relevance to all scientists and clinicians involved in research, development, therapy, risk assessment and regulatory affairs. Internationally respected speakers will address current topics of importance in the agrochemical, cosmetic and pharmaceutical fields and the program will include workshops and poster sessions. Initial enquiries should be addressed to

Dr. Valerie James
PPP Conference
University of Wales
Redwood Building
Cardiff, CF1 3XF, UK
(Tel/Fax +44 (0) 222 874952) or
by e-mail to brain @ uk.ac.cardiff.

Author Index

Numbers written in ***italics*** followed by (A) = Abstracts of the 9th Annual Meeting of the SPS (numbers refer to Abstract number).
Numbers written in **bold** face followed by (A) = Abstracts of the 9th ISBS Meeting (numbers refer to Abstract number).

Subject Index

Vol. 5, 1992

Official Journal of the Skin Pharmacology Society (SPS) and
the International Society for Bioengineering and the Skin (ISBS)

Skin Pharmacology

Journal of Pharmacological and Biophysical Research

Incorporating 'Bioengineering and the Skin'

KARGER

S. Karger
Medical and Scientific Publishers
Basel · Freiburg · Paris · London
New York · New Delhi · Bangkok
Singapore · Tokyo · Sydney

Drug Dosage
The authors and the publisher have exerted every effort to ensure that drug selection and dosage set forth in this text are in accord with current recommendations and practice at the time of publication. However, in view of ongoing research, changes in government regulations, and the constant flow of information relating to drug therapy and drug reactions, the reader is urged to check the package insert for each drug for any change in indications and dosage and for added warnings and precautions. This is particularly important when the recommended agent is a new and/or infrequently employed drug.

Printed in Switzerland on acid-free paper by
Thür AG Offsetdruck, Pratteln

Contents Vol. 5, 1992

No. 1

Reviews

Original Research Articles

No. 2

Review

Original Research Articles

Current Problems in Dermatology (ISSN 0070–2064), **Vol. 20**
Series Editor: H. Hönigsmann, Vienna

Editors: B.J. Vermeer, K.D. Wuepper, W.A. van Vloten, H. Baart de la Faille, J.G. van der Schroeff

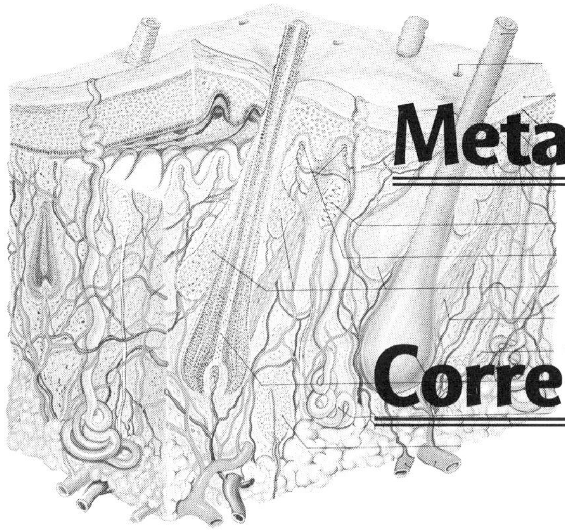

Metabolic Disorders and Nutrition Correlated with Skin

There is much truth in the old adage that the skin is the window into the internal milieu. This volume, based on an international symposium sponsored by the European Society for Dermatological Research, explores the relationship between metabolic disorders, together with their genetic background, and skin disorders and investigates the effects of dietary products on skin conditions. A major part of the book is devoted to improved chemical or genetic understanding of the porphyrias. Among other subjects, many important unsolved problems in clinical dermatology are presented with approaches to their solution, including the role of foodstuffs or their additives in eliciting contact urticaria, atopic dermatitis or systemic contact dermatitis.
Bringing together a wealth of information in a well-defined sphere of dermatological interest, this volume contains rewarding reading for dermatologists and their colleagues in clinical nutrition, clinical chemistry or pathology, genetics and allergy.

Main Headings
Endocrine Function of Keratinocytes
Pancreatic Disease
Thyroid Disease
Lipoprotein Metabolism
Porphyria cutanea tarda
Protoporphyria
Dermatitis herpetiformis
Atopic Dermatitis
Allergic Reactions

Fields of Interest
Dermatology; Nutrition; Metabolism; Allergy, Clinical Chemistry, Clinical Nutrition, Endocrinology, Genetics, Internal Medicine, Pathology

Current Problems in Dermatology, Vol. 20
Metabolic Disorders and Nutrition Correlated with Skin
International Symposium on Metabolic Disorders and Nutrition Related to the Skin, sponsored by the European Society for Dermatological Research, Utrecht, March 1990
Editors: Vermeer, B.J.; Wuepper, K.D. (Leiden); van Vloten, W.A.; Baart de la Faille, H.; van der Schroeff, J.G. (Utrecht)
X + 246 p., 68 fig., 2 cpl., 41 tab., hard cover, 1991
SFr. 250.– / DM 299.– / £ 108.70 / US$ 200.00
US $ price for USA, £ price for UK only (subject to change)
ISBN 3–8055–5361–7

KI91550

KARGER